Plus Size Pregnancy

What the evidence really says about higher BMI and birth

Dr Sara Wickham

Plus Size Pregnancy
What the evidence really says about higher BMI and birth

Published 2023 by Birthmoon Creations

www.sarawickham.com

ISBN: 978-1914465093
Also available as an e-book

Acknowledgements

I want to thank the fabulous people who helped this book to be born, and who supported me on the journey. Huge thanks to Nadine Edwards, Julie Frohlich, Emma Rose, Amy Brown, Becky Reed, Gill Boden, Chris Hackforth, Lucyann Ashdown, Mavis Kirkham, and Debbie Willett.

The complex and specialist nature of this area led me to approach several colleagues and ask them to chat with me or share information about their areas of practice and expertise as they relate to the topics in this book. I have acknowledged and credited them where their words appear directly in the text, but I want to express my appreciation here as well, to Amy Brown, Amanda Burleigh, Ethel Burns, Julie Frohlich, Katie James, Emma Rose, Rachel Reed, Kirsten Small, and also to those who didn't want to be named in the book.

I would also like to thank my colleagues and friends at the Pregnancy and Parents Centre in Edinburgh, Kerri-Anne Gifford and the women and families of the Nottingham Home Birth Group, and all the other women and families who shared their stories with me as I was writing this book, especially as so many of these stories highlight how poorly women with a higher BMI are sometimes treated. This isn't a book of stories, but it is a book that has been inspired by them. Your words and openness in sharing details of what were often difficult experiences have helped me to write a book which I hope will help more women and families to have better experiences of their own. Thank you.

About the Author

Dr Sara Wickham PhD, MA, PGCert, BA(Hons) is an author, researcher and educator who works independently; speaking, writing, teaching online courses and workshops, consulting and creating resources for health professionals, birth workers, writers and others.

Sara has lived and worked in the UK, the USA and New Zealand, edited three professional journals and lectured in more than thirty countries. She has written eighteen books.

You can find and follow Sara online at her website, www.sarawickham.com, where she writes a blog and offers a free monthly newsletter sharing birth-related information. Sara is also on Instagram as @DrSaraWickham

Also by Sara Wickham

Anti-D Explained
Anti-D in Midwifery: panacea or paradox?
Appraising Research into Childbirth
Birthing Your Placenta (with Nadine Edwards)
Group B Strep Explained
Inducing Labour: making informed decisions
In Your Own Time: how western medicine controls the start of labour and why this needs to stop
Midwifery Best Practice (volumes 1-5)
Sacred Cycles: the spiral of women's wellbeing
Vitamin K and the Newborn
What's Right For Me? Making decisions in pregnancy and childbirth
101 Tips for planning, writing and surviving your dissertation

Dedication

This book is dedicated to the memory of two wonderful women and activists: Beverley Beech and Pamela Vireday.

I knew before I sat down to write this book that I wanted to dedicate it to my late, wonderful colleague, Pamela Vireday, also known as Kmom. Pamela was a childbirth educator and size acceptance activist whose courageous, diligent and enduring work on plus size pregnancy helped many women, families, caregivers and researchers. Pamela was a keen unpacker of research and a compassionate advocate. She was for a long time the person who I would turn to for updates on the evidence around higher BMI and birth. Pamela's website is still online, and her words on the next page help explain why this book is so needed.

What I didn't know when I sat down to write this book was that we would lose another wonderful woman, friend and activist just before it was completed. Beverley Beech touched the lives of tens of thousands of women and families in her work as a formidable birth activist and champion of informed decision making. She and I shared many stages, tables, meals, and bottles of wine over the years, as well as our passion for supporting women and families. We also supported each other's writing work. Beverley proofread the last few of my books, often while sitting in my garden, and was planning to do the same for this one. Even in her last weeks, she was asking about the book's progress and sharing her thoughts on it with me, and I can only hope that she would be proud of it (and not find that it contained more split infinitives than she would have allowed!)

"Many websites with information about pregnancy at larger sizes ... publish distorted risk summaries, highlight only the studies with the worst outcomes, tell worst-case scenario stories as if they were everyday events, and imply that complications are inevitable for all fat women. Some even suggest that obesity during pregnancy is akin to child abuse. Not coincidentally, many of these websites are published by weight-loss surgeons, diet companies, or people with weight-loss agendas. Others are published by a medical community (many of whom have ties to the weight loss industry) that has embraced the demonization of fat people."

"What women of size need is more balanced information. They do need to understand possible risks of pregnancy at larger sizes, but they also need to place those risks in perspective and know that many women of size HAVE had successful, healthy pregnancies and births. They need to know that being at risk for a complication does not mean it will automatically happen, and that many women of size never experience complications at all."

Pamela Vireday (2008)

"Am I Allowed? ... The answer to that question is YES! You are. It's your body and your baby and, as with any other medical test or procedure, you have a right to say no, and you should not have to say it more than once. The assumption that one size fits all does not recognise that it might not be right for an individual woman and her baby."

Beverley Beech (2021)

Contents

1. Introduction

Sofia and Ana are identical twins. They are the same age, have the same genetic make-up and are both healthy and fit. They had their first babies within six months of each other and in the same town. But they had very different experiences of pregnancy and birth.

Ana's pregnancy was, in her own words, *"very easy, normal and straightforward."* She had one episode of high blood pressure when she was stressed at work, but says that was, *"as exciting as it got."* Ana gave birth in a midwifery-led unit and she and her baby returned home within a few hours.

Sofia's experience was rather different. From her very first appointment, she didn't get the care she needed. Sofia was offered far more tests and scans than Ana, and found herself under pressure to accept these. She was lectured about her health and choices in a way that she found condescending and inappropriate. At times, she says, she felt judged and shamed. When Sofia expressed an interest in giving birth at the same midwifery-led unit as Ana, she was told this would not be possible. Neither would she be able to use the birthing pool in the consultant unit.

I am happy to tell you that Sofia went on to have her baby the way she wanted, which is how I know her and Ana's stories and am able to share them here. But this was only after she became informed, found more respectful care providers, and was able to access appropriate, evidence-based care. Sofia should not have had to do all these things, and yet the reality is that many women like her are fighting similar battles every day in our maternity care systems.

But why did Sofia have such a different experience from her twin sister, even though they were pregnant in the same town and at the same time? Why did she have such a battle to get the care, place of birth and experiences that she wanted, when it was so much easier for Ana? The two women had similar levels of health and fitness, and in fact Sofia will argue that she is fitter, as she goes to the gym more often than Ana.

But Sofia has a slightly higher BMI, or body mass index, than her twin sister, and BMI is the measure by which people are assessed in order to determine what care they will receive. The difference in the maternity care they received was caused by Sofia being about ten pounds, or five kilograms, heavier than Ana when they went for their first midwife appointment. This put her in a higher BMI category, which meant that her health professionals classified and treated her as 'obese'.

The reality is that, for women with a higher BMI, the path to giving birth in systems of maternity care can be fraught with difficulty. That's because these systems are built around the idea of gauging who is at 'higher risk' and offering those people more tests and a different level of care. And BMI is a key yardstick against which pregnant women are risk assessed. BMI is a crude and questionable measure, and more on that later, and it's not generally used in a careful, nuanced way which takes other individual factors into account. But it's embedded in modern maternity and health care in ways that are affecting more and more of us every day.

Size matters

We live in a world in which size matters. A lot. When a baby is born, one of the first interventions thrust upon it (and deemed important enough to take the baby from the arms of their mother) is the ritual of being weighed and measured.

For months, people will ask a baby's parents, *"what did she weigh?" "How long is he?"* Then we cluck and coo and compare her to her sisters and brothers, to our own babies, to what we see as the average. *"What a lovely big boy." "Oh, you're much daintier than your sister."* Already, the judgement has begun.

During the family's next few encounters with health professionals, they will ask how well the baby is feeding, and continue to weigh and measure the little person. In many countries, the results will be mapped onto growth charts.

In fact, the measuring and mapping already began in early

pregnancy, with tools that attempt to estimate an unborn baby's size and chart its growth, and technologies that aim to predict its birth weight. These technologies aren't particularly accurate, as I will discuss in this book. Despite this, a key pillar of modern health care is focused on measuring our size, weight and shape, mapping those measurements onto charts and graphs, comparing them against averages and man-made 'ideals', and using them to assess, judge and make decisions which affect our lives.

"You're too heavy; you should diet."

"You're too thin; you need to put on some weight."

"You're not entitled to fertility treatment, surgery, or medical help because you're too overweight."

"Your baby is too big/small, you should have an induction."

"Your BMI is over 35, you can't give birth here. You should definitely have more scans and these injections, though..."

A lot of this is rooted in the idea that people with a higher BMI are more likely to have health problems. Therefore, risk screening is used to identify them so that health professionals can offer advice, care, and intervention. But there's a problem. The ideas that underpin this approach aren't based on robust evidence, which means the approach may not be effective. In fact, it's worse than this, because there's growing concern that it may be causing harm, on a number of levels.

What's the problem?

When we look at the evidence, it turns out that the focus we place on size, weight, and BMI impacts many different people, of all ages and stages. It's not just those with a high BMI. People who are deemed to be underweight or who have a low BMI also experience negative consequences from the assumptions and lack of evidence to support what happens in this area. The societal emphasis on size and shape pervades the media and social media and affects everyone in some way.

But, while I am just as concerned about those problems, this book has been written for a very specific group of people.

It is for and about women like Sofia. Women who have a higher BMI and who are trying to navigate maternity care and make decisions about what's right for them.

I know that this book is very much needed. Having been involved in maternity care for thirty years, I've seen how the measures, guidelines and approaches taken towards weight and BMI are increasingly used to risk assess, categorise, label, restrict, and control pregnant women who have a higher BMI. According to Public Health England (2019), 50% of all women are overweight or obese at the start of pregnancy, so the policies, guidelines, beliefs, and recommendations relating to BMI and the treatment of larger people now affect around half of those seeking maternity care in England.

Over the past few years, the care experienced by larger people has worsened. Size discrimination and fatphobia are, sadly, all around us. Women who have a higher BMI feel pressured to accept more interventions during pregnancy and birth (Blaylock *et al* 2022), and report feeling shamed and stigmatised by the approach taken (Knight-Agarwal *et al* 2016, Jones & Jomeen 2017, Relph *et al* 2020, Blaylock *et al* 2022). This wouldn't be acceptable or ethical even if the pathways and practices were evidence-based and led to better health. But, as I mentioned above, much of what is being offered to women with a higher BMI isn't evidence-based. Moreover, some of the beliefs that underpin this approach are mythical, racist, misogynistic, and just plain wrong.

Are there some things that might be helpful to do or know about if you're living in a larger body? Yes. It's totally up to you whether you decide to accept or decline them, of course, but there are things you might decide you want when you read the evidence. It's appropriate that health care providers offer tests and interventions when they are effective and based on sound evidence. But, as I will discuss in this book, many of the guidelines underpinning the offers of tests and interventions are based only on opinion. Some practices, restrictions, decisions, and care pathways are rooted in fear, profit, power, or tradition rather than focused on optimising health and wellbeing. And that's not okay.

For example, as I was writing this book, media stories highlighted conflicts of interest wherein a pharmaceutical company promoting weight-loss injections was found to be, *"...paying the salaries of staff on NHS obesity teams and financing the launch and redesign of services,"* and funding the people chairing guideline-making bodies (Das & Ungoed-Thomas 2023). A row broke out about the Royal College of Midwives' (RCM) partnership with a commercial weight loss company (Donnelly & Taylor 2023). Many RCM members took to social media to express their concern that evidence was being ignored. They reported that referrals and personal data were being handed over from health services to a commercial company. They spoke of their fear that profit was being put above the protection of women's physical and mental health.

This is not, by the way, a criticism of anyone who finds weight loss programmes, drugs, or diets useful. Some people want to engage with them and find them effective or helpful. That's fine. But much of what is being offered to those with a higher BMI isn't evidence-based. Restrictive dieting only works for a small minority of us (and then not always in the long term). Many of the tests, programmes, and interventions have negative long-term consequences, and these approaches often involve blaming and shaming, which undermine confidence and damage health. There are, however, other approaches that are worthy of attention, and a bigger picture that many people don't know about.

Like so many areas, it's complex. Certainly more complex than those who pontificate about the so-called obesity epidemic would like you to think. And I will tell you upfront that, even though I wasn't totally new to this area when I began to write this book, I was surprised and shocked by some of what I learned. You might be too. But we need to examine the evidence and question what is happening. The key to resolving the problems that exist in this area is to help women and families to understand the evidence and the issues, so they can make the decisions that are right for them.

Introducing myself and this book

Just so you can get a sense of who I am and what the tone of this book is going to be like, let me introduce myself. Having enjoyed a career in independent midwifery, academia and information, I now focus on analysing medical research and writing books. I love to explain research and statistics to people who don't like maths. I'm also a plus size woman, and have been all my life. I've seen prejudice and fatphobia in health care for decades. So I understand the pain, frustration, and injustice of being judged, labelled and put into a box based on the application of a racist, sexist, nineteenth century, one-size-fits-all index that isn't based on evidence. More on that in chapter two.

Over the past few years, I have heard from hundreds of women, families, care providers, and birth workers who are deeply concerned about the BMI-focused approach. It's stark listening and reading. I've met women who have felt shamed, triggered, and guilty at every appointment, and this is also the finding of researchers who have studied this area (Blaylock *et al* 2022). I've heard endless stories of people who have been given poor advice, or been told that they must or must not do certain things. Some, like Sofia, have had their preferences denied or been prevented from making informed decisions simply because of their size or shape.

Most of these people would have been open to considering a different path or additional intervention if it were truly warranted and demonstrably advantageous for them or their baby. But, when they asked, the evidence wasn't forthcoming. Some were fobbed off. A few said they didn't dare ask, for fear of being further shamed. I've talked to women who were told they had gestational diabetes and then instructed to follow a diet that didn't feel healthy to them. I've met women who would have been happy to have interventions that are proven to be effective but found that care providers didn't understand the evidence and couldn't see beyond their BMI, shape, or weight.

Women and families want and deserve better answers to their questions. Is there a direct link between BMI and health? Are women with a higher BMI genuinely at higher risk, and, if so, of what? Is it a good idea to meet an obstetric anaesthetist in pregnancy if you're planning to give birth in the birth centre? Won't that undermine your confidence? What are they assessing anyway? Why are you being offered aspirin? What's low molecular weight heparin, and is there good evidence that it will help? Do these things have downsides? Is your baby really at risk because you have more fat in your pelvic area? Is induction of labour really preferable for larger women? Do bigger women genuinely have a problem labouring, or is that professional prejudice? And why are some larger women told they can't use a pool in labour, and what can you do to turn that around?

I'm going to look at the evidence for all of these things and many more. I also bust some myths, and share with you the advantages of having a higher BMI, both in general and in relation to pregnancy and birth. The 'fat is bad' message is so powerful and profitable that we don't tend to hear about these advantages, but they do exist.

This isn't just about challenging the incomprehensibly profitable diet industry, though. It's about helping you feel more informed. If you're a parent-to-be, I hope this book will help you understand your options and the evidence. If you're a health care provider or birth worker, I hope you'll use this evidence to support those you care for, and challenge the elements of the current approach that aren't evidence-based, supportive, helpful, or kind. Because what's often happening in this area isn't any of these.

In chapter two, I'm going to explain a bit about the history of our beliefs and the evidence in this area, unpacking the notions of diet culture and BMI, and looking at why our current approach to weight, health and dieting is problematic. Chapter three looks at BMI and maternity care. It offers an explanation of the approach that is taken and will give you a deeper understanding of some of the key ideas that underpin modern maternity care, including how our attitude to risk shapes the way in which larger people are treated. A key element of this approach is the idea that larger women and their babies are more at risk of some unwanted outcomes. In chapter four, I dive into the evidence about those outcomes, and will show how the claims made about risk and BMI are actually not quite as straightforward as we are told.

In chapters five to seven, I discuss the evidence and the wider issues relating to the various tests, interventions and restrictions that are offered to those with a higher BMI during pregnancy, labour and birth, and after birth. Each chapter ends with a few tips from women, families, midwives, and birth workers. Chapter eight draws the book to a conclusion.

As is the case with a few of my other books, there is some deliberate repetition of information now and again. That's not because I or my editors have missed things. It's because, having written several books over many years which help women and families to understand the evidence on different topics, I'm aware that some people will be reading sections in a hurry, while under pressure to make a decision. I hope that those of you who have the time to read this book like a novel will forgive the occasional repeat, for the benefit of those who only have time to flip through it to find what they need.

Finally, I want to offer my usual reminder that there is no right or wrong path here. As with so many areas, it's important that you can weigh up the evidence, consider the wider picture, understand that the things that are offered can sometimes cause harm as well as good, and get a sense of where there are gaps in our knowledge. My aim is to explain the situation and the evidence so that you can pick the path that's right for you and your family.

Sara Wickham. Wiltshire, England. Summer 2023.

2. BMI, diet culture and myths

> *"For most of human existence, no one dreamed of restricting their food intake to lose weight. Getting enough food was the main concern, and plumpness signified prosperity and well-being. Fat on the body meant higher social status, a better chance of weathering famine and disease, and a greater likelihood of fertility. Thinness meant poverty, illness and death."* (Harrison 2019: 17).

If you are living in a high-income country today, and you turn on a television, computer or phone, or even just have a chat with another person, it is highly likely that you will encounter one or more stories about the problems of overweight and obesity. Such narratives, and the worrying statistics that are used to underpin them, are hard to avoid, not least because they are a mainstay of news agencies. Today, I have seen discussions about how governments should be doing more, or doing different things to solve the problem. I've scrolled past articles promoting weight loss injections, and ignored adverts for recently published books which offer yet another new approach to weight loss or healthy eating.

It's almost impossible to escape conversations about the 'obesity epidemic', although if that word bothers you then let me assure you that I won't be using it more than I have to. People are concerned that we are getting larger, and there are lots of theories as to why this is. Thousands of research papers are published every year, and those of us who live in larger bodies are constantly urged to eat less, eat better, lose weight, exercise, and accept tests, interventions and criticism because we are deemed to be 'at risk' as a result of the size, shape and weight of our bodies.

I probably don't need to tell you how stressful it is to be on the receiving end of this. It's also incredibly confusing to try to work out what one is supposed to do about it, especially when there is so much contradictory information out there, and a new diet or approach at every turn. Things get even more confusing for those who try the diets or programmes and find they don't work, or that they stop working after the first bit of weight loss. Some find that they put weight on, and can't understand why, because they followed the plan.

I'd like to assure you that, if any of this resonates, you're not alone, and you're not imagining it.

As is the case in so many areas, what we watch, read, and encounter in everyday media and conversation is only part of the story. If you dig deeper into the issues and the evidence, as I started to do a few years ago, you find scientists, social scientists, and researchers whose work is adding to our knowledge and helping to tell a deeper, more nuanced story.

Some researchers suggest that the 'fat is bad' narrative isn't universal, and "*...the majority of the world's cultures had or have ideals of feminine beauty that include plumpness*" (Brown & Konner 1987). Others show that fatphobia isn't new (Hagen 2020). But our current ideas about weight, health, and size have become established in the last 150 years or so, during periods of history characterised by industrialisation and standardisation (Harrison 2019). One example of how this still affects us today is that, before the industrial era, our clothes were custom made. The rich would have a seamstress or tailor, while the poor would sew their own outfits. Mechanisation in clothing manufacture led to standardised dress sizes and the need to measure ourselves (Harrison 2019). I think lots of us will be glad that we don't have to sew our own clothes but, as Harrison explains, this wonderful shift also had a negative consequence: "*body shame and comparisons with your friends*" (2019: 23).

This is just one example of why we need the bigger picture. I'm certainly not advocating throwing out medical research and the valuable things that we can learn from it. But it's important to remember that there are other perspectives, and some of them show that what we have come to believe isn't the whole truth. That's what I want to explain in this chapter.

A word about the word obesity

I'm very aware that words like obesity and overweight are insulting, offensive or triggering to some people, so I try to limit their use to situations where I'm directly quoting research or in which meaning would otherwise be lost.

I would also love it if I had been able to write this book without using the phrase 'normal weight' when comparing outcomes between women with a high BMI and those with a BMI of 18.5 to 24.9 kg/m^2. That's the narrow range which is considered 'normal' or 'healthy' within western medicine. I'll come back to why this is a problem when I define BMI. I have avoided such terms except when I am directly quoting others or where a critical point might otherwise get lost.

There's another important thing to know about words like these, especially 'obesity' and 'overweight'. They are simply adjectives used to describe someone's size, either according to their BMI or in comparison to some mythical average person. While many organisations, people, books, and adverts tend to use the word obesity as if it describes a medical condition, it actually does not. A medical condition is an illness, injury or disease, and obesity is none of these things.

Researchers have pointed out that the notion of obesity is a human construct; *"a culturally produced idea with social effects"* (Ellison *et al* 2016: 4). I learned while researching this book that the term 'morbid obesity' was created by a doctor, Howard Payne, in an attempt to increase the demand for the bariatric (weight loss) surgery that was his specialty. Coining this term *"was an ingenious way to frame bariatric surgery as a necessary and even lifesaving operation, because labelling people's body size as morbid makes it sound like they're about to drop dead. By creating a new class of larger bodies that were supposedly near death because of their size, Payne made the strictures of diet culture a little more oppressive"* (Harrison 2019: 38-39).

The idea that obesity is a medical condition in itself can also be harmful, especially when the messages that I'll discuss in this chapter are all around us. The mass media tends to present obesity statistics as *"a disaster and warn[ing] of a looming global health catastrophe"* (Gard & Wright 2005: 17). However, this catastrophising isn't helpful or effective, and there are concerns that this approach can cause harm.

Looking at the bigger picture

I've already explained that there's a bigger picture here. A growing body of research is giving us good reason to question some of our culture's current beliefs about weight, size, BMI, and what we should be doing about these. It's just as important to consider what the research doesn't show. I've found no evidence, for example, that having a higher BMI in itself causes any disease. Having a high BMI is associated with having a higher chance of some conditions for some people, but it doesn't cause anything. There just aren't simple, straightforward relationships between BMI and health.

Some of the scientists and social scientists who question the western medical idea that living in a larger body is inherently risky have pointed out that our modern cultural beliefs about weight, health, BMI, and dieting are part of the problem. Social scientists, nutritionists and other experts in this field have created a term to describe this set of beliefs: they call them 'diet culture' (Harrison 2019).

The beliefs of diet culture include the idea that being fat is risky, that there are 'good' and 'bad' foods, and the importance of exercise for weight loss. It's not only health professionals who hold these beliefs, but much of society too. In fact, the beliefs and effects of diet culture are all around us, in such a marked and pervasive way that we often may not even notice them. We are constantly exposed to ideas about food, weight, body shape, calories, dieting, eating, and drinking. For instance, lots of us believe that weight is directly related to what someone eats, and this idea feeds other beliefs, such as the one where larger people are thought to be greedy, weaker and have less self-control. But these ideas are not evidence-based. In fact, it takes rather a lot of self-control and willpower to diet for years, which is what many larger people have done, sadly often without long-term success.

Yet these ideas have taken root. They prioritise weight and shape over health and have negative consequences, including stigma, mental health problems, body dysmorphia, and disordered eating (Bacon 2008, Harrison 2019). This way of thinking ignores the evidence showing that our weight is largely out of our control (Caro *et al* 1996, Kojima & Kangawa 2005, Bacon 2008, Izquierdo *et al* 2019, Wolrich 2021).

Ironically, believing and following the ideas of diet culture can lead to ill-health. We now know that our bodies will fight low calorie diets by adapting and cutting back on the resources that go to other body systems, such as immunity and cellular renewal. It's not just that diets don't work. They are actively bad for our health (Bacon 2008, Harrison 2019, Wolrich 2021).

I don't have room in this book to explain every aspect of the science relating to weight, attempted weight loss, diet culture, and the wider issues raised by these. Those deserve (and have) entire books written about them, and the science is ongoing. Nor will I discuss the weight loss drug industry, which excites some people, concerns others, and raises key political, ethical and social questions. Instead, I want to briefly explain why it's valid to question the modern approach to weight, weight reduction and related topics, from a number of angles. That's because having an understanding of the wider picture is key to thinking about how these issues affect childbearing women and families.

The first thing that we need to understand and question is one of the most fundamental beliefs of western medicine and diet culture. It affects anyone seeking health or maternity care. That is, the idea that an index developed 200 years ago in a small sub set of people is a good measure of health today.

The body mass index (BMI)

BMI is used throughout the world as a way of assessing people's body size. In mathematical terms, someone's BMI is their weight in kilograms divided by their height in metres squared. But there's no need to even get a calculator out because BMI is deemed so important today that there are literally thousands of web pages, apps and charts that will do the sums for you.

Health-related organisations have chosen arbitrary cut-off points to put people into categories according to their BMI (WHO 1995). In most countries, a BMI of 18.5 to 24.9 kg/m^2 is defined as 'normal' or 'healthy,' and anyone whose BMI is 18.4 kg/m^2 or less is said to be 'underweight'. People with a BMI of 25.0 to 29.9 kg/m^2 are considered to be 'overweight', and anyone with a BMI of 30.0 kg/m^2 or above is said to be 'obese'. There are then different classes of obesity, and the following list shows all of these categories.

Underweight - BMI 18.4 kg/m^2 or less
Normal/Healthy - BMI 18.5 to 24.9 kg/m^2
Overweight - BMI 25 to 29.9 kg/m^2
Obesity class I - BMI 30 to 34.9 kg/m^2
Obesity class II - BMI 35 to 39.9 kg/m^2
Obesity class III - BMI 40 kg/m^2 or higher

In some countries, different cut-off points are used for certain groups. For example, World Health Organization (WHO) researchers suggested lowering BMI cut-off points to trigger public health action for people of Asian descent. They argued for labelling people with a BMI of 23–27.5 kg/m^2 as overweight and those with a BMI ≥27.5 kg/m^2 as obese (WHO 2004). These suggestions are controversial and haven't been fully adopted.

Whichever cut-off points are being used, the range of 'normal' is narrow. Moreover, the use of the words 'normal' and 'healthy' to describe this narrow range gives the incorrect idea that people in other categories (which is most of us) are 'abnormal' or unhealthy. This isn't true and it can be harmful. It's another example of how myths, theories, and stigma have become embedded in research, guidelines and conversation.

Within systems of maternity care, BMI is seen as a critical piece of information. The BMI cut-off points above are used to assign a risk status and trigger the tests, interventions, and restrictions that I will discuss throughout this book. As one's BMI increases, so do the tests and interventions offered. But where did the idea of BMI originate, and why do many people now believe that it is problematic?

The history of BMI

The unpleasant truth about BMI and why it's a poor standard by which to measure our health begins in 1832, with a Belgian mathematician called Adolphe Quetelet. Monsieur Quetelet was interested in many subjects. He corresponded with Florence Nightingale, Francis Galton, Karl Marx, and Goethe, among other prominent people of his time. Quetelet founded the Brussels Observatory and directed it for many years. He loved the idea that we could learn useful things by measuring populations, and was fascinated by the idea of the average man. For him, though, this meant the ideal or average man in an aesthetic sense, an idea associated with Leonardo Da Vinci's depiction of the 'Vitruvian Man.' It's important to know that, for Quetelet, this was an academic and artistic exercise; he wasn't commenting on health at all. Quetelet created an equation that combined body weight and height into an index which became known as 'Quetelet's index'. We now know that same index as the body mass index, or BMI.

Quetelet's index didn't catch on immediately. But, as time passed, more attention was paid to possible relationships between size, shape, weight, and health. The insurance industry thought there might be a correlation between weight and life expectancy, and began publishing tables relating to what they saw as the relative risk in this area (Association of

Life Insurance Medical Directors 1912). These tables were crude and they didn't work well, so people tried to improve them. In fact, we now know that the reason they didn't work well was because there isn't a direct correlation between size and health (Harrison 2019). Several other ways of assessing people's 'fatness' were developed, but none was considered particularly effective until an American physiologist named Ancel Keys came along.

Ancel Keys is a controversial figure. Some of his work is questionable to say the least, but it still has a big influence on the ideas that hold strong today. Keys came up with and promoted the idea that saturated fat should be replaced by polyunsaturated fat. He contradicted those who were concerned about the effect of refined sugar on health, thus delighting the sugar lobby. Keys was responsible for K-rations (WWII US army food portions now known to have been lacking in nutrition and often described as monotonous) and the Mediterranean diet. His ideas have been highly influential in what we now call diet culture.

Most importantly for our purposes, Keys rediscovered and promoted Quetelet's Index, which he called the body mass index. He declared in 1967 that BMI was the best means of measuring relative body weight (Keys *et al* 2014). Keys' justification for this assertion was a study that he and his colleagues carried out. It involved gathering together data collected from *"epidemiological studies related to coronary heart disease"* (Keys *et al* 1967: 4). The included countries were Finland, Greece, Italy, Japan, the Netherlands, the USA, and the area formerly known as Yugoslavia. The populations studied were almost entirely white, male, middle-class, and middle-aged.

We have long known that BMI differs with age, sex, and race (Gallagher *et al* 1996), so BMI is another medical construct introduced by middle-class white men that doesn't take into account Black and Brown people, women, people older or younger than the study participants, or anyone who doesn't fit the white man's idea of 'average' or 'ideal'. BMI is therefore a two hundred year old index that was originally about attempting to measure the average white man for artistic purposes (Cryle & Stephens 2017) and it isn't evidence-based.

Sadly, the racism doesn't end with BMI being based on the measurements of white men. Strings (2015, 2019) shows how fatphobia is rooted in racism, and is *"a means of using the body to validate race, class, and gender prejudice."* Justin & Jette's (2022) work confirms that *"21st century efforts to medicalize fatness, by diagnosing 'obesity' via the Body Mass Index (BMI), has aided in the construction of 'obesity' as an 'epidemic' (Evans and Colls, 2009; Gard, 2008; Gard and Wright, 2005; Lupton, 2012). These efforts marginalize Black women, in particular."*

The cut-off points that determine what category someone is put into are arbitrary and have changed over time. BMI is known to be inaccurate in people who are older, or who are particularly tall or short, and it has been shown to have low sensitivity and specificity as a screening test (Rothman 2008). Sensitivity and specificity refer to how accurate a screening test like BMI is at working out who may have a problem without over-diagnosing too many people who don't have a problem. There's more on this in chapter five. BMI has been repeatedly shown to be a poor screening test on both counts.

To be honest, BMI doesn't have a lot to recommend it, except that it's simple and already in mass use. Despite this, the use of the flawed notion of BMI as a way of measuring someone's health, risk, and entitlement to certain types of care continues almost unabated. Unfortunately, the fact that BMI is simple and universal makes it really hard to overturn, because anyone seeking to challenge it needs to convince millions of medical practitioners and other people that it's of no use. When you consider that BMI is also a core component of some of the key myths of diet culture, and thus at the root of a number of ideas that are making a lot of people a lot of money, it may be easier still to understand why something so flawed is still in everyday use.

Let's look at those myths next.

The myths and messages of diet culture

This is an overview rather than an extensive review of the myths and messages of diet culture. I'm hoping, in this section, to give you a summary of the problematic myths that our culture has adopted about weight, weight loss, and health, as well as the messages that are transmitted, as a basis for moving on to discuss the issues that exist in maternity care. If you'd like more detail on any of these topics, I've tried to reference papers and books that are fairly accessible.

The myth that BMI is a proxy for health

The first myth of diet culture is that someone's BMI can be used as a proxy for their health status. As I already noted, the relationship between BMI, size or weight, and health status is not straightforward (Bacon 2008, Harrison 2019, Treasure & Ambwani 2021, Wolrich 2021). Many people believe the *'being fat is bad as it leads to poor health'* message that has pervaded our culture for decades, but that doesn't mean that it's based on sound evidence.

There is some evidence of correlations between being larger and having poorer outcomes in some areas of health (Guh *et al* 2009), but there are a couple of important caveats. First, the results in studies which show that larger people have a higher chance (risk) of a particular health outcome than people of lower weight often aren't as significant as they are made to sound. That's because it's important to look not just at the relative risk (X is twice as likely as Y) but at the absolute risk as well. And, when you dig into the numbers and look at the absolute risk of something, the risks are often so small to begin with that a doubling of the risk still leads to a really small chance of something. Absolute risk doesn't make good headlines though, so that's why those who want to sell stories or diet clubs will focus on relative risk. There's lots more on risk reporting in maternity care in chapter four.

Another important issue to consider is that evidence

showing that two things are associated or correlated is absolutely not the same as evidence showing that one of those things causes the other. Both might, for instance, be caused by something else. Having a higher BMI might be caused by another health factor. In fact, when it comes to higher weight people and poorer health outcomes, there are a number of things that could be causing both. It is vital that we remember the potential health impact of socioeconomic factors such as racism, poverty, stress, and misogyny.

Factors such as whether someone smokes or moves their body regularly have a far greater impact on health than BMI. Research doesn't always account for, look at, or mention these. In fact, the one-size-fits-all, population-based approach increasingly taken by those promoting a western public health model doesn't account for individuality at all. We need to stop trying to categorise everyone according to one factor (for example BMI) and instead look at overall health.

It's also important to address some of the myths about weight and food intake. Do some people have poorer health because they are larger as a result of eating poorly and not taking care of themselves? Undoubtedly. But some people are larger for other reasons too. As Bacon (2008: xxi) clarifies, *"body weight might be a marker for an imprudent lifestyle in some people, but its role in determining health, particularly when compared to regular activity, is grossly exaggerated."*

It's entirely possible to eat what our culture perceives as a healthy diet and still have a higher BMI, or to eat far more than everyone else in the family and have an average or low BMI. I also want to acknowledge how confusing it can be to try and work out what a healthy diet actually is, because so many groups try to persuade us that theirs is the best. There may be no 'one-size-fits-all' answer to this either, and a lot of people are now questioning the unhelpful idea that there is such a thing as a universally healthy diet, or so-called 'good' and 'bad' foods.

So is everyone who is larger unhealthy, and at higher risk? No. Is it appropriate to send women like Sofia on a different journey just because of a slightly higher BMI, which might be accounted for by muscle or being especially short? Not at all. Is it more acceptable if someone is much larger, and has a very high BMI? Still no. BMI isn't a proxy for health. We need to look more widely at the health of individuals, and pay attention to the fact that, *"...many researchers over the years have recommended that BMI be discarded as an outdated and ineffective tool for measuring health."* (Harrison 2019: 36). For more on this, see Bacon (2008), Harrison (2019), or Wolrich (2021).

Weight stigma and the messages of diet culture

I want to pause my discussion of the myths of diet culture briefly to mention one of the key consequences of diet culture: weight stigma. This is also known as weight bias or weight-based discrimination, and it refers to the stereotyping, mis-treatment, and discrimination that many people who weigh more or have a higher BMI experience.

Weight shaming can occur in overt, direct statements about body size or health and as covert messages, for instance someone rolling their eyes and huffing about needing to get a different piece of equipment, raising their eyebrows, pulling faces, or casting their eyes at someone's body as they try to sit in a chair that isn't size-friendly. Sometimes, stigmatisation and shaming are used intentionally, in an effort to try to humiliate people into performing the behaviours that will supposedly lead to weight loss. Such ideas are embedded in many medical guidelines, recommendations and practices.

Weight stigma and discrimination transmit some of the key messages of diet culture: *fat is bad, and people who are fat are lazy, greedy, undisciplined and not as worthy*. Those messages are untrue, unevidenced, unpleasant, and harmful (Puhl & Heuer 2010, Anon 2020, Kuehn 2020, Rubino *et al* 2020). Researchers running the Health At Every Size® study (Bacon 2008) quickly also showed them to be incorrect:

"[In] contrast to the negative stereotype of the lazy and undisciplined fat person, everyone in this group had exhibited

tremendous determination, strength of character, and willpower in their persistent attempts to lose weight." (Bacon 2008: 2-3).

Weight stigma doesn't work. It can cause physiological stress (Muennig *et al* 2008), and it poses numerous negative consequences for psychological and physical health (Puhl & Heuer 2010). Somewhat ironically, the consequences of weight stigma include obesity (Vadiveloo & Mattei 2017, Harrison 2019). A systematic review of 33 studies found that

"Weight stigma was positively associated with obesity, diabetes risk, cortisol level, oxidative stress level, C-reactive protein level, eating disturbances, depression, anxiety, body image dissatisfaction and negatively associated with self-esteem among overweight and obese adults." (Wu & Berry 2018: 94)

As Tomiyama *et al* (2018) also show, the effects of weight stigma have been shown to occur independently of weight. In other words, these findings can't be explained away as being the consequence of someone's weight or size.

Weight stigma is found at many levels of our culture. It is embedded in the mass media (Kite *et al* 2022, Heslehurst *et al* 2022), where *"the dominant discourse* [is about] *viewing overweight and obesity as an individual responsibility and overlooking systemic factors"* (Kite *et al* 2022). Researchers have shown that social media platforms are full of non-experts who glorify weight loss and present the idea that thinness is preferable to being larger (Minadeo & Pope 2022). But genuine subject experts are often no better. Weight stigma has also been shown to be endemic in health, medical and maternity care (Wray & Deery 2008, Furber & McGowan 2011, Mulherin *et al* 2013, Christenson *et al* 2020, Incollingo Rodriguez *et al* 2020, Hurst *et al* 2021, Nagpal *et al* 2022).

One reason that fatphobia, weight stigma, and the negative consequences of diet culture are endemic is because so many people believe these ideas. The myths are also perpetuated by partners, friends, family members, lay birth workers, and others. It's important to recognise that this isn't just a health professional and maternity services problem. It's a much wider cultural problem.

"I thought I would protect myself by hiring a doula. But she was every bit as fatphobic as some of the midwives. She used softer language but the message was the same: you're not okay as you are, it would be better if you changed. Constant little comments and tips about food, as if I didn't know what healthy eating looked like. I hate [how] even seemingly supportive people think it's okay to tell you that their idea of health should be yours." (Polina)

Polina's words also help explain why it's hard to research weight stigma. It's because some of our deepest beliefs about weight, size, and related issues are so deeply embedded into our culture that most remain unaware of them (Harrison 2019). Yet these messages are everywhere.

In 2020, a multi-disciplinary group of international experts published a joint consensus statement with recommendations to eliminate weight bias (Rubino *et al* 2020), which was reported in the medical literature (Kuehn 2020, Anon 2020).

"People with obesity commonly face a pervasive, resilient form of social stigma. They are often subject to discrimination in the workplace as well as in educational and healthcare settings. Research indicates that weight stigma can cause physical and psychological harm, and that affected individuals are less likely to receive adequate care. For these reasons, weight stigma damages health, undermines human and social rights, and is unacceptable in modern societies." (Rubino *et al* 2020)

Weight-based discrimination was also acknowledged as a significant problem in a 2021 House of Commons Committee report (UK Parliament 2021), in which the chair, Caroline Nokes, said, *"The use of BMI as a measure of healthy weight has become a kind of proxy or justification for weight shaming. This has to stop."* (Mahase 2021)

Sadly, this call has been largely ignored. There is no shortage of evidence that weight stigma, anti-fat bias, and fatphobia damage health. However, as with many of the areas where we are now learning that modern culture and western medicine have got it wrong, there is a lack of willingness from those who benefit or profit from the current system to challenge or change it.

The myth that we should attempt to lose weight

The next myth of modern diet culture is the cultural expectation that those who live in larger bodies or have a higher BMI are expected to take responsibility for this and to follow recommendations to 'correct' their weight. As Wray and Deery (2008: 227) explain, *"under the rhetoric of 'health', a large body size has come to be symbolic of self-indulgence and moral failure."*

Yet we know that higher BMI can be the result of stress and the inequalities of racism, social class, misogyny, poverty, and prejudice. These are often interrelated (Marmot 2020). Even if it were acceptable to tell someone what to do with their own body, research shows that weight and size are multifactorial in origin. These factors include genetics (Logel *et al* 2015, Saqlain *et al* 2022), stress, the microbiome, endocrine (hormonal) function (Ochner *et al* 2013), metabolic health and others (Caro *et al* 1996, Kojima & Kangawa 2005, Bacon 2008, Izquierdo *et al* 2019, Wolrich 2021). These are not all within the control of the individual. Weight and size can also be affected by several different health conditions, including thyroid disease and cancer.

If that weren't enough, evidence increasingly shows that deliberate weight loss isn't even possible for most people in the long term. We have also seen that the problem isn't a lack of willpower. I noted above that the people in Bacon's (2008) research were highly motivated and exhibited tremendous strength of character and determination. I have also explained the harm that stems from an approach that posits being larger as a moral failing which needs to be rectified.

People gain weight in situations and ways they often have little or no control over, yet they are then blamed, shamed, and expected to rectify this by following the rules of diet culture. But, as I will explain in the next sections, they can get caught in a cycle of attempted weight loss on diets and programmes that aren't effective but can negatively affect their health while helping others profit.

There is no 'should' about it.

The myth that diets are effective

Contrary to popular belief, there is good evidence that restrictive diets and weight loss programmes are not effective or beneficial and may do harm (Stunkard & McLaren-Hume 1959, Wing & Jeffrey 1979, Crawford *et al* 2000, Bacon 2008, Bacon & Aphramor 2011, Fildes *et al* 2015, Harrison 2019, Treasure & Ambwani 2021, Wolrich 2021). Restricting calorie intake often leads to something called the yo-yo effect, where people lose weight and then regain it, sometimes with a little more on top, which puts them back in the hands of the weight loss companies. The extra weight that some people gain each time they diet may, some scientists and researchers think, be the result of their body panicking because it thinks it's being starved. This is why quite a few people get bigger over time, despite trying many different diets.

Researchers are beginning to understand why a restrictive approach doesn't work. Scientists have now shown that:

"Weight gain is relatively easy, but the human body is just not designed to support weight loss. This means that reversing weight gain habits will do a pretty good job of preventing weight gain, though they may not result in weight loss." (Bacon 2008: 22)

One reason why significant calorie restriction isn't effective as a long-term weight reduction strategy for about 95% of us is because our bodies have cleverly learned over many millennia to recognise any food restriction as a form of famine (Bacon 2008, Wolrich 2019, Harrison 2019). It is somewhat ironic, as Bacon (2008) points out, that those of us alive today are likely to be especially good at retaining and putting on weight. Thank you, natural selection! We literally have the genes for weight gain because, until a few hundred years ago for those living in high-income countries, the ability to put on and maintain weight in a famine was necessary for survival.

Unfortunately, there is no sign that anyone is going to stop recommending weight loss plans and programmes, and for good reason. A 2021 report calculated that *"the global market for weight loss products and services should grow from $254.9* *billion in 2021 to reach $377.3 billion by 2026"* (Research and Markets 2021). Many of these programmes are based on a 'repeat customer' business model. You are warmly welcomed to the group and programme, and praised for having made the decision to prioritise your health. You are well supported to lose weight (which is possible for many people if you restrict your diet in the short term; it's keeping it off in the long-term that's the problem) and waved off when you achieve your target with cheers of congratulations. However, the people behind such programmes are often well aware that the human body has evolved to respond to food restriction in a particular way, which is to say that it will now do whatever it can to help you regain the weight that you lost. Even as those who profit from these programmes smilingly watch you walk away, they may know it's only a matter of time before they will welcome you (and your purse or wallet) back into the group to begin the cycle again.

The myth that losing weight leads to better health

It's important to address the myth that weight loss leads to better health, because there isn't good evidence for this either (Bacon 2008, Harrison 2019, Treasure & Ambwani 2021, Wolrich 2021). In fact, I already shared evidence that dieting – especially 'yo-yo' dieting, which is basically the business model of slimming groups that I just described at the end of the previous section – can worsen our health.

An issue of particular concern in relation to pregnancy is that dieting often means restricting nutrient intake. Women have an increased need for vitamins and minerals (for instance calcium) in pregnancy. Restrictive dieting before or during pregnancy may lead them to lack these vitamins and minerals, which can then be exacerbated when their body prioritises their growing baby's need for these. Many women report being praised for weight loss, but at what cost does this occur? If someone has lowered their BMI but has then become vitamin deficient and is experiencing postnatal depression or exhaustion because they removed an entire food group from their diet, is that a 'win'? We must consider the bigger picture.

This is a complex area to research, partly because of some of the myths I've already talked about. When we try to carry out studies on the effects of having higher body weight in the context of a society that discriminates against larger people, it's hard to separate possible effects of having higher body weight from the harmful effects of dieting, and being exposed to weight stigma. Research into pregnancy and childbirth doesn't often look at long-term health, or mental health. It doesn't help that many of the so-called 'obesity experts' behind the current recommendations and research funding have ties to the diet industry, slimming groups, and pharmaceutical companies who make and sell weight loss and other drugs offered to those with a high BMI (Kotaska 2018, Brown 2019, Harrison 2019, Das & Ungoed-Thomas 2023). Parker and Bero (2022: 1) showed that *"over 95% of members of the US dietary guideline committee (2020) had financial links to the food or pharmaceutical industries."*

Finally, much of the work that has been done around weight and health has focused on the relationship between BMI and the chance of developing diseases which tend to occur in later life. Just like Quetelet's and Keys' work, a good number of the research studies that underpin the modern medical approach to BMI and health have focused on older people, most of whom are white men. So how is this relevant to the health of women who are pregnant and giving birth in their twenties, thirties or forties? It's vital that we question the effect of dieting before or during pregnancy, and whether this has long-term effects on women's health. This is just one reason why some people wonder if it would be better to 'go back to the drawing board'; to reconsider what health looks like if we take BMI and the myths associated with it out of the equation, and go back to the principles of good health rather than continue to use an index based on the dimensions of middle aged white men that wasn't ever intended to measure the health of anyone, let alone pregnant women.

Metabolic health

Many of those who have questioned the value of BMI as a way to assess health point out that it doesn't correlate with indicators of metabolic health. But what does that mean?

'Metabolism' is a word used to describe all the chemical processes that happen inside our bodies in order to help keep us alive. We are all made up of many millions of cells, and those cells need to be nourished by food, water, vitamins and minerals. Metabolism is the breaking down of food and anything else we ingest (such as vitamins or supplements) into smaller particles, after which some of these smaller particles are then rebuilt into substances that our body needs. If someone is metabolically healthy, all of the complex body processes that make up their metabolism are working normally. Metabolic diseases, such as diabetes mellitus, occur when something isn't quite right.

In diabetes, for instance, the amount of glucose (sugar) in the blood is higher than health experts consider to be optimal. This may be because the pancreas isn't able to produce insulin, which is what happens in Type 1 diabetes. People with Type 1 diabetes need to take insulin throughout their lives. Type 2 diabetes is a condition in which the body either isn't producing enough insulin for the metabolism to function in a healthy way, or where the cells aren't reacting to insulin in the way that they should. There is also a condition called prediabetes, which is where blood glucose levels are a bit higher than normal, but not high enough to be classed as diabetes. You may also have heard the term gestational diabetes, which describes high blood sugar that occurs during pregnancy. I'll discuss that further in chapters four and five.

Some health professionals and researchers believe that we should focus on metabolic health instead of BMI, because metabolic health – which is assessed by measuring things like blood pressure and blood sugar – is a better measure of how our bodies are functioning. BMI doesn't correlate with metabolic health (Lebovitz 2003). It's true that people who are larger are a bit more likely to have diabetes or other metabolic disease compared to those with a lower BMI (Ganz *et al* 2014, Gray *et al* 2015, Guo *et al* 2021, Teufel *et al* 2021). However, some people with a high BMI are metabolically healthy, and plenty of people with an average or supposedly healthy BMI have poor metabolic health (Lebovitz 2003).

There are other ways of measuring health and wellbeing. These include considering whether someone is strong, fit, flexible and able to do things they enjoy and that enable them to live an independent life. None of these things are directly related to BMI either. Researchers are also looking at how some people tend to lay down more fat around their internal organs than others and that this kind of fat (and not necessarily the kind that lodges on one's thighs, bum or tummy, which is also, by the way, the kind we tend to lay down in pregnancy) is the kind that is associated with health issues in later life (Kang *et al* 2012, Xiao *et al* 2018). It's sometimes referred to as 'fat on the inside' and, while it's not something I'm going to discuss in this book, it's easy to look up if you want to know more. Some people argue that we should use waist-to-height ratio instead of BMI (although this would be hard in pregnancy) and call on those who devise guidelines to look more closely at the evidence and consider better ways of measuring health (Ashwell & Gibson 2016).

These are just a few examples of how our use of BMI as a way to measure health is being challenged, including from within the medical community and weight loss industries. In fact, we need to know a lot more than we currently do, and there are plenty of avenues to explore. For instance, evidence shows that health effects differ between those genetically predisposed to being larger and those who have a higher BMI as a result of environmental factors (Ojalehto *et al* 2023). However, in order to find out more about these areas, we need more researchers to put aside the existing myths and be willing to explore ideas outside of their current belief systems and modes of thinking.

When BMI is a particularly illogical measure

I want to add a couple more examples about how illogical it is to use BMI as a measure of health, because these further show how our approach isn't based on evidence or common sense. I'm going to keep saying throughout this book that it's important to take a wider perspective and to look at things in the context of each individual person, and here's why.

First, BMI tells us nothing about where someone's weight comes from. Many world-class athletes have a high BMI, with rugby players and weightlifters being good examples. Muscle weighs more than fat. This also means that someone who decides to be more active and undertakes muscle-building activity is likely to find that their weight and BMI go up, rather than down. This is just one more reason why it's important to take a wider view of what we mean by health. It's also a reminder that, if you are athletic or have well-developed muscles because you do a lot of physical work or (like Sofia) you go to the gym, you may want to take BMI-related recommendations with an even larger pinch of salt.

As I was writing this book, Lead Midwife Emma Rose pointed out to me how breast size can also have an influence on BMI as *"the difference between one BMI category and the next can sometimes be five pounds. So a generous bosom can make all the difference, which is another way in the context of BMI in which women are at a disadvantage compared to men."* Again, we know that women and men lay down fat differently (Gallagher *et al* 1996), but BMI is based on measurements of men.

Second, relying on BMI alone can lead people to make illogical decisions. Women with a higher BMI sometimes find it hard to negotiate using a hospital birth pool. This is because hospital staff need to consider how someone would be helped out of the pool if an emergency arose. I'll discuss this further, including what you can do about it, in chapter six. But it's not logical to use BMI as a means of gatekeeping birth pool access.

For example, Annie is five feet (150cm) tall and has a BMI of 35. She weighs 82kgs, or 180lbs. In some areas, she would be told that she couldn't use the birth pool because of her higher BMI. But Bonnie faces no such restriction, because she has a BMI of 29. Bonnie also weighs 82kg, but she's five foot six (168cm). Her BMI is lower simply because she is half a foot taller than Annie. But she weighs exactly the same to anyone needing to help her out of the birth pool.

The same thing happens when we take a higher cut-off point, say a BMI of 40. Charlie and Dionne both have a BMI of 40. Charlie is four foot eight (142cm) and weighs 82kg, or 180lbs, just like Annie and Bonnie. Dionne is five foot eleven (180cm) and weighs 132kgs, or 290lbs. Despite having the same BMI, their height and weight are very different. I'm not saying it's acceptable to restrict Dionne's use of the birth pool because she weighs more, by the way. I'm using this example to show how, just as we need to consider the absolute risk of something happening rather than just looking at relative risk, we also need to look at someone's actual weight, height and other characteristics, not just an index measure like BMI. It's just common sense but, as one of my teachers used to like to remind us, common sense is unfortunately not that common. That seems to be particularly the case in bureaucratic systems which run on rules and recommendations that are encased in guidelines and encoded in compulsory paperwork, and in computer systems that refuse to negotiate.

Other things are important too. In the birth pool example, we might also consider someone's function, fitness, state of health, or ability to move. We could take into account who else will be there, and whether appropriate lifting equipment is available. It's also relevant to consider how often women become unconscious in birth pools, and I'll cover all of that in chapter six. Sometimes we shouldn't be measuring anything, or at least not using those measurements as a basis for imposing restrictions.

But whatever the relevant factors are for the situation at hand, there are multiple reasons why we shouldn't be using BMI as the sole way of measuring someone's health, as a marker for whether we perceive them to be at higher risk, or as the basis for making decisions about their care.

The advantages of being plus sized

No, you didn't misread that heading. People with a higher than average BMI have some health advantages, both generally and in pregnancy. These benefits aren't widely publicised, however. This is probably because both western medicine and our culture are so keen to sell us the *'fat is bad'* myth, and to berate, shame and punish larger people for what they see as a self-caused problem.

There is a phenomenon called the obesity paradox and, while I don't love its name for reasons already mentioned, I do love that we know about this. I also love that our growing knowledge of this area is serving as a fly in the ointment of diet culture, getting some researchers to look beyond their existing beliefs, and perhaps helping to reverse some of the negative effects of weight bias and fat shaming.

The term 'the obesity paradox' was coined to describe some research findings which challenge the belief that fatness always equates with ill health. For example, larger people are more likely to survive and have better recovery from cardiovascular and cerebrovascular disease, some types of cancer, and strokes (Brzecka & Ejma 2015, Antonopoulos & Tousoulis 2017, Carbone *et al* 2017, 2019, Elagizi *et al* 2018, Belladelli *et al* 2022). In simple terms, people researching these areas think that stored fat may help protect and nourish the body as it undergoes healing, or encounters medical treatments that have side effects.

It's just as hard to research the obesity paradox as it is to research the effects of size on other aspects of health, though. That's because of the multiple factors at play and, again, the weight bias that exists in medical research. When reading about the obesity paradox, I was struck by the tone of many researchers. It is as if some of them cannot and do not want to believe their own findings. There is a sense that, as they write, they are thinking, *'there must be another explanation, because being fat is bad, I just know it is'*. The fact that it is even described as a paradox points to how illogical and unexpected it is as an idea. But such an idea is only unexpected and illogical within the context of a culture where fatness is viewed and judged so harshly that any advantages of this are greeted with shock and surprise by fatphobic researchers.

I suspect that even more findings that show benefits to having a higher BMI are not being published because weight-biased journal editors and researchers do not want to highlight them. The existence of the obesity paradox, like so many of the ideas, studies and findings that I have shared in this chapter, challenges their fundamental worldview. As history shows, people often rail against, mock and challenge new truths for a good while before the volume of evidence finally gives us no option but to accept them (Kuhn 1962).

But the obesity paradox exists, and we are learning more about it all the time. While writing this book, I chatted with gynaecologists who are wondering whether larger women have different experiences during and after menopause. This is because oestrogen is stored in fat. Some think one reason women put on weight around their tummy in perimenopause is to store oestrogen. They call it a 'lifebelt'. That's a really different way of thinking from the 'fat is bad' approach.

I also talked with an orthopaedic surgeon who explained that, while there seem to be advantages and disadvantages to weighing more when it comes to bone health, he doesn't see as many larger women for certain types of surgeries.

"It's the frail, bird-like little elderly ladies that I get concerned about, not those with meat on their bones. To some extent, as long as they are well-nourished and getting some exercise, larger women seem to have stronger bones. It makes sense physiologically, it's just not aligned with what we generally believe about the ill-effects of higher weight." (Tom)

Being larger also brings a few advantages when it comes to childbirth, but I'll save that good news for later. First, let's look at how systems of modern maternity care approach the issue of BMI.

3. BMI and maternity care

For a good few years, health and medical organisations and many of those who work for them have believed that obesity is a condition that (a) negatively affects health and (b) is potentially modifiable. As you'll know from chapter two, those things aren't actually true, at least for the majority of us. But, as more people are now realising, beliefs that underpin government policy aren't always true or evidence-based. The House of Commons Women and Equalities Committee called upon the British government in 2021 to review its obesity strategy and ensure it was evidence-based (UK Parliament 2021). The Committee urged Public Health England to stop focusing on BMI as a measure of health and instead adopt the Health at Every Size® (Bacon 2008) approach. This hasn't happened. The few changes that have been made don't reflect the evidence or the recommendations of the Committee.

This isn't really surprising. The recommendations which underpin health and maternity services are often not based on robust evidence (Prusova *et al* 2014, Wickham 2021a, 2021b, Reed 2022). Recommendations are influenced by the values of those who write them. In our culture, obesity is seen as a problem which needs to be prevented and treated, so this has become an important focus within health policy and strategy. Committees have sat, experts have shared their thoughts and beliefs, targets have been developed against which we can measure our progress in reducing obesity, and a vast amount of money is available to those who set up programmes, groups, research, and interventions to try to address, reduce, and prevent it. As long as they don't challenge the prevailing viewpoint or the tenets of western medicine.

The strategic focus placed on obesity by governments and medical organisations around the world is the reason that anyone seeking health care with even a slightly raised BMI is likely to encounter unsolicited obesity-related conversations and weight loss interventions. Pregnant women are especially likely to experience these, and on multiple occasions. This is because pregnancy is seen as an ideal time to undertake health promotion and launch health interventions, because people are particularly open to them (Atkinson *et al* 2016).

From the perspective of those making health policy at a population level, this makes a lot of sense. Most pregnant women are generally healthy, which means they might not otherwise go to see a health professional. If you are trying to find a way to catch up with youngish, healthy people and instil health messages and interventions, pregnancy is a good time to do so. Pregnancy is also perceived as a time in which people are highly motivated to form healthy habits, because they want to do what's best for their baby. This may not be ethical, but it is common. So it is perhaps inevitable that organisations such as Public Health England (2020a), the Australian Institute of Health and Welfare (2022a), and many others around the world have made pregnancy a strong focus in their obesity reduction strategies.

But this approach is at the root of some of the problems that plus size women face. There is a real tension between a public health approach and one which sets out to meet and treat women as individuals who may or may not want to follow population-level recommendations or to be the recipient of numerous public health messages that are not necessarily evidence-based. Sanders *et al* (2016) described this as like coming up against *"a wall of information."*

Not a new problem

The idea that our approach to the care of larger women is questionable at best and harmful at worst is not a new one. In 2009, I wrote an article for a British midwifery journal which ran a special issue to look at issues relating to larger women. I talked about the 'naming, blaming and shaming' that was occurring in maternity care (Wickham 2009). I was driven to write it by a number of things, not least of which were the experiences of the women in my care.

I was also responding to the recent publication of another midwifery journal whose obesity-themed issue ran with a cover depicting a towering sandwich. This, as I wrote at the time, *"led to an epidemic of rolled eyes amongst those who are passionate about trying to help and support women in ways that are non-judgemental and evidence-based"* (Wickham 2009). It reinforced the untrue message that anyone who is larger than average has become that way by eating 'unhealthy' food. There was lots of judgement but no real understanding of the complexity of this area: the harm done by weight stigma; the false assumption that there is a direct relationship between what one eats and what one weighs; and ignorance of the multiple factors at play.

It wasn't as if we didn't know better. The journal for which I wrote contained papers asking similar questions, and my article drew upon and cited some of the work that was happening in maternity care at the time. This included studies like those by Wray and Deery (2008), who had looked at the medicalisation of larger body size and highlighted myths such as the idea that being larger was the result of *"self-indulgence and moral failure."* We already knew at that point from Hunt and Symonds (1995) and Nyman *et al* (2010) that larger women receiving maternity care felt judged, over-scrutinised, and humiliated by caregivers and others. Even some of those who used terms such as *'obesity epidemic'* acknowledged that the issue was complex and that the best way forward may not be the existing approach (Bick 2009).

Sadly, the questioning of the status quo and the growing body of evidence offering another viewpoint didn't stop the juggernaut that was the modern medical idea that plus size pregnant women needed to be pathologised and treated differently. In fact, efforts were made to publicly shame some of us who were speaking out, because not only did we have the audacity to question the status quo, we also dared to do so whilst inhabiting larger bodies ourselves.

In the decade and a half that has passed between then and now, we have seen a proliferation of guidelines, screening tests, recommendations, and restrictions aimed at women with a higher BMI. As a midwife colleague wrote to me while I was writing this book:

"I'm increasingly disturbed by the stories of the treatment of healthy fit pregnant women and what appears to be 'plus size BMI' stigmatisation. I've been around long enough as a midwife to remember not having to do any BMI measures at booking-in. 'Plus size' (I don't even like this terminology!) women were having much more enjoyable pregnancies and ordinary care and very happy outcomes too. There were also plenty of home births I and colleagues attended for women of 'plus size' back then." (Kerri-Anne)

These changes are due in no small part to the proliferation of guidelines which exhort health professionals to offer extra screening tests and interventions to women with higher BMIs, and to restrict them from situations which are perceived to be risk-laden. It's the contents of those guidelines that I'm going to examine throughout the rest of this book. Before I do that, I want to explain a few things about guidelines, evidence and the approach taken in maternity care so that anyone who is new to the area has some background information.

Guidelines, recommendations and evidence

In most countries, maternity care is informed by written guidance; documents that guide practitioners to know what to do or offer to people in different situations. Many countries now have guidance for the care of women with a higher BMI, who are *offered* screening tests (for instance weighing someone to calculate BMI), additional tests and interventions in the hope that these will help reduce the chance of problems.

My spelling out of what guide means and my emphasis on the word offered in the previous paragraph is deliberate. It's important to know that guidance only tells doctors and midwives what to offer. Guidelines are not a mandate and you are not compelled to go along with any of them. Although I acknowledge that these tests and interventions don't always feel as if they are presented as an offer, nothing is compulsory. If this is something you would like to know more about, please see my book, *What's Right For Me? Making decisions in pregnancy and childbirth* (Wickham 2022).

In theory, because we live in an era where it's deemed important to base practice on evidence, the guidance is based on the findings of good quality research studies. Research is gathered and analysed by people deemed to be experts and used to form recommendations about what should be offered.

In theory.

When one analyses the guidelines, however, a problem is quickly revealed. As I've now mentioned several times, they are not always reflective of the actual evidence. They are instead often based on outdated and unevidenced myths, opinions, and assumptions. A systematic review and quality appraisal of international clinical practice guidelines (CPGs) on weight management showed that *"45% of CPGs were appraised as poor quality, 32% as moderate, and 23% as high"* (Harrison *et al* 2021). The researchers also found that the recommendations were *"highly variable between guidelines,"* and their analysis uncovered *"significant ambiguity in existing guidance."*

Similar results were found by a later study by Kominiarek *et al* (2022) who explained that, *"evidence-based guidelines for peripartum care are lacking."* They carried out a large review of obesity-related recommendations and tools, and found that *"the recommendations for peripartum care for persons with obesity are based on limited evidence and few practical tools for implementation exist"* (Kominiarek *et al* 2022).

If we take just one guideline as an example, we can see this problem clearly. I will discuss elements of the Royal College of Obstetricians and Gynaecologists (RCOG) Green-Top Guideline on the *'Care of Women with Obesity in Pregnancy'* (Denison *et al* 2018) throughout the next few chapters, but a quick glance at it reveals that, out of 63 recommendations, only three are based on grade A evidence (which is a systematic review, meta-analysis or high quality randomised controlled trial). Another 17 of the recommendations are based on grade B or C evidence (which includes good-quality cohort and case control studies). The majority of the recommendations (68%) are graded as D-level evidence, such as individual case reports or the opinion of those who were on the committee. Kominiarek *et al* (2022) also found that a third of the recommendations (13 out of 39) in the guidance they looked at were based on expert opinion rather than research evidence.

But expert opinion is just the theories and beliefs of a group of people. They may be open- or closed-minded. They may or may not be woman- or person-centred. They may have strong beliefs for or against many things, and these beliefs will inform their opinions and thus what ends up in the guidelines. For example, a guideline based on the opinions of a group of privately educated, narrowly-read, conservative, middle class white men who personally and professionally profit from diet culture and are only interested in short-term outcomes is likely to come up with a different opinion-based guideline to that of a more diverse and open-minded group which is focused on long-term outcomes and includes people who will be personally affected by the guideline.

Sometimes, those who compile the guidelines are well aware of their shortcomings, but this doesn't stop them being used to underpin care. A good example in this instance is the NICE (2010) guidance on *'Weight management before, during and after pregnancy.'* A read of the documents attached to this guideline clearly shows that many of the statements are not supported by evidence. In several cases, even when evidence is cited, it is of poor quality and hasn't taken the full picture into account. Review notes attached to the guideline acknowledge that some of the recommendations in the document are known to be incorrect and that some sections were deemed to need a 'refresh' back in 2014. At the time of publishing this book, around a decade later, those updates had still not been undertaken.

This is an international problem. A similar lack of evidence and reliance on opinion can be found in guidelines created by the American College of Obstetricians and Gynecologists (ACOG 2021), and the Royal Australian and New Zealand College of Obstetricians and Gynaecologists (RANZCOG 2022). A senior obstetrician has detailed the shortcomings of previous RANZCOG guidelines (Teale 2020), yet the issues he raised have not been addressed in more recent versions.

"There are disparities in these guidelines and some provide limited advice on key aspects of care. It is notable that almost all of the recommendations in the RANZCOG 'Management of Obesity in Pregnancy' statement are graded as 'consensus based'. This highlights a paucity of high-level evidence for mitigating the risks, and much of the advice contained within the statement is common sense." (Teale 2020)

Comparing these international guidelines highlights yet another issue. Kominiarek and Chauhan (2016) compared BMI-related guidelines from five countries, and found *"substantial differences in the recommendations."* Given that I am an advocate for individualised, midwifery-led care, I do not think that we should be reliant on guidelines for all aspects of care. Putting this aside for a moment, the fact that the guidelines relating to this topic are contradictory confirms that the evidence on which they are based is debatable. If recommendations were based on abundant, robust and clear evidence, and on science rather than opinion, the documents from different areas of the world would be similar to each other. But they are not.

Challenges that women with higher BMI face

The lack of evidence for the care that is offered is only one of the issues in this area. I have mentioned that many studies show how dissatisfied plus size women are with the way they are treated within maternity services (Wray & Deery 2008, Furber & McGowan 2011, Mulherin *et al* 2013, Jones & Jomeen 2017, Thorbjörnsdottir *et al* 2020, Heslehurst *et al* 2022). There are a few other interrelated problems that women with a higher BMI report encountering during maternity care. These are things that I will be discussing throughout the rest of this book, and I am going to list them here and then use the rest of this chapter to explain the underpinning issues a bit more, especially for those who are new to the area.

The key issues faced by plus size women are:

- Experiencing weight stigma and fat shaming.
- Being inappropriately labelled as 'high risk.'
- Being told they need to lose weight and perhaps attend groups to help them manage their weight.
- Being denied some types of care/experience.
- Being told they need additional tests and interventions.
- Experiencing care provider doubt in their body's ability to give birth physiologically.

The problem with risk and risk labelling

Risk is a key focus in maternity care. Almost every test, intervention, and restriction recommended for people with a higher BMI is based on claims that larger people have more chance of experiencing unwanted outcomes than those with a lower BMI. In other words, larger people are perceived to be at higher risk, both during childbirth and more widely.

Risk is a scary word. It can evoke fear and, if someone tells you that you or your baby are at high risk of something, it can feel terrifying. Many women have told me they were scared into agreeing to a test, drug, restriction, or procedure that they did not want, and that they later regretted. That's why I explain the concept of risk and the data relating to different outcomes in so much detail in my books. It's also why I advocate for using the word *chance* instead of the word risk. It means the same thing, but it takes the fear away, which can help in decision making.

The word 'chance' is also a useful reminder of the way in which life isn't predictable or controllable. Some people might like to think that we can control nature, but that's not how it works. Yes, we can do some wonderful things thanks to science, but there are no guarantees, and we can't control, prevent or change everything. That includes some aspects of our own situation. It might well be that you have a slightly higher chance of experiencing something because of things like your age, family history, or BMI on a given day, but these aren't things you can change, and we now know that labelling people as 'high risk' can be misleading and even harmful.

In chapter four, I will use data from research studies to explain why people with a higher BMI aren't necessarily 'at high risk' in the way that they are often told they are. But before we get to the statistics, I want to explain why the risk labelling used in maternity care is so problematic.

Medical intervention is amazing when people experience accidents, have emergencies, or develop treatable diseases or conditions that can benefit from surgery. In such situations, intervention can prevent harm and sometimes be lifesaving. There are a few situations in maternity care that are genuine emergencies, in which we can fairly say that someone is at high risk of a problem if we don't intervene, and quickly. For example, if a woman is bleeding heavily and the usual methods of stopping bleeding don't work, that's a genuinely high risk situation. Similarly, if something goes wrong during a caesarean or someone has a blood clot in their lung, those are high risk circumstances.

But being labelled as 'high risk' is very different from having an actual disease or problem. Falling out of a tree and breaking your arm is an actual problem. Being told you're more at risk of breaking a bone if you walk around a park than if you stay sitting on the ground on a picnic blanket is risk labelling. It may well be true, but your chance of falling over is very low, there may be risks to sitting on the ground, and if all we ever did was to sit on picnic blankets and worry about risk then our lives would look quite different.

It's the same in maternity care. When health care providers label a pregnant woman as being at 'high risk,' they don't mean that she has an actual medical problem. They usually mean that she has one or more markers - which can be things like her age, BMI, means of conception, blood pressure, blood type, blood sugar level, or something in her previous experiences - which they have identified as risk factors.

Some of these risk factors are based on data showing that women in one group have a higher chance of experiencing a situation than women in another group. Others, as I noted above, are based just on opinion. But whatever their basis, there are a few things to know about this. On the one hand, most of the people labelled as being 'at high risk' won't experience the problem that they've been told they might. On the other hand, some of the people who didn't get the 'high risk' label will experience it. The actual chance of a poor outcome may not be very high, and we'll come to that in chapter four. When you look at the data, it often turns out that 99 per cent of those labelled as 'at high risk' don't experience the problem, which begs the question of why the focus is put on the one per cent of occasions when things go awry rather than on the 99 times they go right.

In health care, claims about someone's risk status are often based on population data. Research findings often show that people in one group have a higher chance of experiencing something than people in another group. The defining feature of the group which has the higher chance of a problem (for instance, older women, those who have had three or more babies, women with a high BMI) becomes the basis for assigning a risk status and telling practitioners who to offer tests and interventions to do so.

This is a crude way of assessing health, which only works at a population level. If you're working for a government and trying to make decisions about where to allocate limited resources, it might be justifiable - from an ethical perspective - to use these data as the basis for your decisions. When you're an individual looking at your options, things can look very different. One question that is always worth asking is what your actual chance of experiencing a problem is, and not just whether a person in group A is at higher risk than a person in group B. We call actual chance the absolute risk, and I'll come back to this in chapter four as well.

It's also important to look at the downsides and risks of whatever you're being offered in the hope of preventing the problem. That includes the benefits of what you're missing out on by accepting an intervention, test or restriction. If, for instance, you accept electronic fetal monitoring in labour, you may not be able to move around as well, or to use a shower, bath, or birth pool. That could affect the progress of your labour, which can in turn affect whether or not you're offered drugs to speed up labour, a caesarean or instrumental delivery. This is a concrete - and sadly all too common - example of how the risk labelling itself can be the cause of the intervention that leads to the outcomes that women are told they are at risk of. A focus on risk can also, as women often tell me, *'steal the joy'* from your experience of pregnancy.

In Blaylock *et al*'s (2022) study, *"Some of our participants described being told they were 'at risk' or had a high-risk pregnancy but not being told how much greater their risk of a poor outcome was. This was particularly the case with risk factors which were unmodifiable at the time of pregnancy such as having a high BMI or suffering from a pre-existing health condition. This failure to contextualise risk derives from how risk is calculated from population-level epidemiological studies and extrapolated and applied to the individual in a clinic setting."*

Weighty conversations

If you haven't personally experienced maternity care, you may not know that the challenges faced by plus size women can begin from the moment they enter a booking appointment and continue through subsequent consultations.

"My weight dominated every conversation held with every single medical professional and led me and my partner to be absolutely convinced we wouldn't bring the baby to term. We were told repeatedly that the birth would be difficult, I wouldn't cope and

that there would be complications. I was told to have an epidural at the first signs of labour as I would def need emergency intervention so it made sense to do it at the beginning as I wouldn't be able to control myself enough once the labour had started to do it later on…. I was almost convinced I wouldn't be bringing my baby home and even didn't do things like put up a cot." (Survey respondent, Blaylock *et al* 2022)

It's so awful to read words like this, but I include them because they illustrate how harmful the current approach is. Because the idea that being heavier makes one 'high risk' is embedded in maternity care guidelines, it's difficult to get through pregnancy, birth and the postnatal period without your weight being made a focus of conversation and care.

Some midwives, doctors, and other health professionals also prefer to avoid weight-related discussions, but this can be difficult when they are embedded in maternity care policy. Health professionals are sometimes made to tick a box to state they have calculated your BMI and discussed this with you.

One study (Atkinson *et al* 2017) found that some midwives didn't want to raise the issue of weight, or were very careful to present the offer of referral to weight management services as an option which could be declined. Yet the study's researchers criticised the midwives, saying that this led to inequitable services. They discussed ways in which midwives could be persuaded to refer more women to such services.

Because many care providers understand that people often don't want those conversations, and are told to seek permission before discussing weight (PHE 2020), you will often have to do no more than hold up your hand as a 'stop sign' or say that you are not interested in having that conversation. It can be less stressful than you might fear, and I offer tips on how to manage this in chapter five.

It is possible, of course, that you may welcome these conversations. If so, great. Some authors state that women value weight loss conversations and interventions during and after pregnancy (McParlin *et al* 2019, Tyldesley-Marshall *et al* 2021). Yet in my experience, and in other studies (Blaylock *et al* 2022), many plus sized women report finding conversations about their weight to be intrusive, unwanted, and potentially offensive. So why the discrepancy?

The answer is probably fairly simple, and it can show us something very important about how research studies are conducted and why we should always treat research findings with caution. Imagine that there are 100 women in a room and we ask them to move to the left if they would welcome a conversation about their weight and to the right if they do not want this to happen. Let's say that half of the women move to each side of the room. Now, we ask a new question. We ask the women to raise their hand if they would be willing to participate in a research study in which they will be asked questions about their weight. We explain that, in the study, they will be weighed, have their body measured, and then undertake weight loss interventions. Do you think there will be an equal number of hands up on each side of the room?

I don't. I think it's far more likely that the women on the left-hand side who wanted to talk about their weight would agree to participate in a study compared to those who didn't want to talk about it. So when researchers ask the women who agreed to participate in the study how they feel about weight loss conversations, they shouldn't be surprised to find that a high proportion of participants either don't mind or actively wanted these conversations. We know that a high number of women decline to join weight loss studies (Bick *et al* 2020). Those who didn't want to have those conversations are probably less likely to have agreed to be in the study in the first place. The sample in these studies is therefore biased towards those who are comfortable discussing their weight.

There are other factors at play as well, and one of these is that women may feel pressured into saying what they think the researchers want to hear. That's particularly important in a culture which constantly tells people that they should want to be slimmer, and where many women feel under pressure to be 'good' mothers and to do the 'right' thing, even when there's no evidence behind it.

Measuring, monitoring, intervening, restricting

While some organisations no longer recommend weighing at every visit (NICE 2019a), most women will be asked to step on the scales at some point in pregnancy; usually at their first (booking) visit with a midwife.

I am spelling this issue out for a very good reason. Weighing is itself a screening test. If you step on the scales, your BMI will be calculated and used to determine the care that you will be offered. But here's the important thing:

It's your decision whether to be weighed or not.

That said, the measuring of someone's actual weight (not their BMI) can sometimes be important if they are going to have certain medications, notably anaesthetic and some forms of pain relief. I will come back to this later. In almost every other healthcare setting, the act of weighing someone is done because either their absolute weight or their BMI is going to be used, likely without their consent or knowledge, to place them into a risk category. As I showed with Sofia and Ana's stories in chapter one, a few pounds or inches can make a significant difference to someone's experience. Then, as you now know, it is BMI that determines what tests, interventions and restrictions will be offered or applied.

Some women respond to inappropriate BMI-related restrictions by taking matters into their own hands. Adjoa describes feeling *"so angry that I was told that I couldn't have her [my baby] at the birth centre because of my BMI. Well, I wasn't going to the consultant unit so I gave birth at home. They couldn't ban me from my own bath."*

The extra tests and interventions can have a significant impact on the experience of pregnancy and birth, as Kelsey explains: *"They wanted to monitor me, then there were these looks they shared because they couldn't hear him as I was larger. So they went to put some clip on his head,* [and I said] *well no, actually, because you can't give me a good reason to do this in the first place. But I just wonder how labour would have been different."* (Kelsey).

The NICE (2019a) antenatal care guideline acknowledges that some women do not wish to have their BMI calculated.

But be aware that this is not the case everywhere, and some health professionals will estimate your weight even if you decline. This can also happen with size-friendly caregivers, because of the way the system is set up, or as a result of local pressure. In the UK, for instance, the recording of a woman's BMI at booking is one of the minimum standards for the NHS' Maternity Services Data Set (MSDS). Data are anonymised and used to commission services, monitor outcomes, and address inequalities. UK Hospital Trusts have to collect a certain amount of data in order to meet quality standards. Similarly, in Aotearoa New Zealand, midwives are unable to book women into state funded maternity care unless they input a BMI onto a central computer system. They cannot get past the screen without inputting a mandatory number. These examples further illustrate just how deeply ideas about the importance of BMI are embedded into health care.

In such situations, some midwives tell me that they guess, make a number up, or ask the woman what she wants them to put. This is a good example of what Mavis Kirkham (1999) describes as 'doing good by stealth', where midwives find ways to resist the dominant, medicalised birth culture. However, as Kirkham (1999) herself pointed out, while it can make a big and important difference for individual women at that time, doing good by stealth doesn't in itself do anything to challenge the system or change the status quo for others. It's also important to know that even a made up or guessed BMI that is recorded in your medical notes can still impact upon your care. Sadly, there aren't always good solutions, and these are points that need to be raised and discussed with those organising care.

Racism, poverty and disadvantage

It is also important to understand that certain groups of women are at even greater risk from the BMI-focused approach of modern maternity care. While the current approach to weight, BMI and the care of larger people needs addressing across the board, and while women are more disadvantaged than men, there is also a racist element to the modern approach which further disadvantages Black and Brown people. But inequalities are often not taken into account when guidelines are drawn up.

I've explained that the basis of BMI is racist, and many of the studies that I looked at for this book either haven't included the experiences and outcomes of Black and Brown people, or they haven't separated out the data so that we can learn things that might be useful. As Justin and Jette's (2022) study of Black women's experiences illustrates, the dominant obesity discourse (by which we mean the way our culture values thinness and talks about size and related issues such as health and weight loss) doesn't take into account cultural differences and the way in which size, shape and fitness are differently interpreted by different groups.

I also already noted that BMI was based on measurements of white men. But we have the further problem that, while Black (Flegal *et al* 2005, Ogden *et al* 2015, Public Health England 2020b) and indigenous (Australian Bureau of Statistics 2019, Ministry of Health 2021) women have the highest rates of obesity in some high-income countries, the current approach doesn't take into account cultural differences, the impact of colonisation and racism, or how Black and indigenous women are differently disadvantaged.

Another example is that some databases show that South East Asian women are more likely to have a BMI which categorises them as underweight (WHO 2004). This means they have a higher chance of experiencing outcomes such as a serious perineal tear (Gurol-Urganci *et al* 2013), and of being more compromised if they bleed a lot after birth.

In some cases, Black and Brown women are offered yet more intervention, without evidence of benefit and without being able to make informed decisions about whether these interventions are right for them. In 2021 in the UK, moves were made at a national guideline level to consider offering induction to Black and Brown women at 39 weeks without any evidence that this would make a positive difference to outcomes (Wickham 2021a). Over the past few years, I've also received a disproportionate number of queries about evidence for blood thinning medicines from Black and Brown women and their caregivers compared to white women. And while writing this book, I was deeply concerned to hear from Black and Brown women who told me that they had been offered an additional ultrasound scan, described to them as 'an ethnicity scan'. There is no evidence that additional scans are of benefit. However, as I discuss in chapter five, we know that scans carry risks and downsides. A key concern is that they lead to additional interventions, which carry further risk.

As in so many areas, recommendations are being made without evidence, whilst key areas such as mental health are not being given the attention they deserve. When one considers that Black and Brown women and babies are at higher risk of morbidity (illness) and mortality (death) than their white counterparts (Knight *et al* 2022), it might seem odd that I'm questioning these things. Surely we want to do everything possible to help improve outcomes?

Well yes, we do. Which is why we should be especially careful before offering tests and interventions which have costs and potential downsides as well as potential benefits and which may limit women's access to the types of care which are known to make a positive difference. Rather than claiming that the increase in adverse outcomes faced by Black and Brown women with higher BMI has anything to do with the size or shape of their bodies, we need to address the poorer health care that both Black and Brown people and people in larger bodies receive. It is important that we look at genetic differences, where these exist, but it's even more important to take a much wider view in considering how we can tailor appropriate, individualised health care that might improve rather than worsen outcomes.

Another group that is of particular concern is women who are living in poverty. These women also experience poorer outcomes (Knight *et al* 2022), and not enough attention is being paid to how current frameworks of care mean that they are additionally disadvantaged. As just one example, even if nutritional advice can be shown to be beneficial, it is not helpful to those who cannot afford or cannot gain access to the kinds of foods that are often recommended. Nutritional advice is also often given without taking somebody's cultural norms into account. These might include food preferences, foods that they avoid, and issues such as festivals, ritual fasting and cultural beliefs. Other potentially important cultural norms also include what kinds of foods someone is used to cooking and eating, where they shop, who is responsible for shopping and food preparation, and what is possible within the context of their family and life.

It's clear that we need to do better in these areas.

Amy's story

The issues discussed in this book don't only apply to those who fall into the category of having a higher than average BMI. Yes, that is my focus for the majority of this book. But weight stigma, fatphobia, the myths of diet culture, and our society's obsession with size, shape and appearance affect us all, whatever our size, shape or weight. I was reminded of this when I chatted about this book with my friend and colleague, Amy Brown. Amy is a professor who has herself written about the research relating to BMI, and I quote some of her work in later chapters. Amy shared her pregnancy story with me for this book to help illustrate how the beliefs that many people hold about size and weight can affect the experience of pregnancy, birth and maternity care, not just for plus-sized women, but actually for all of us.

"I had hyperemesis [severe vomiting] *for each of my three pregnancies, all the way through. So by the time I was getting weighed around that 12 week point, I had lost loads of weight, so I had a healthy BMI, and then I just did not put on weight through that pregnancy hardly, because I was vomiting numerous times a day, all the way until the end.*

"And the amount of praise I got from some midwives and health professionals! I remember one telling me I was lucky because I wasn't putting on weight, and it was because I was vomiting every hour and, as you can imagine, losing significant amounts of weight. Luckily because my BMI was around 24, 25 when I got pregnant, I still had some weight that I could theoretically lose, but nobody was concerned about that at all. Because the baby was alright and because I wasn't being hospitalised, they would just comment on how great it was.

"And of course that then always had the reaction, probably combined with the hormones of breastfeeding, that I would rapidly gain weight after the birth, keep it on whilst I was breastfeeding and then of course I was chastised for gaining weight. Even when, with the third baby, I developed a thyroid problem, and the weight gain was due to the thyroid problem, it was seen the other way around ... that, somehow, I must just be overeating. Even though the thyroid diagnosis was right there in front of them.

"My BMI only went up to 32 at the most, yet still you get that message; you're damaging your health, you need to lose weight, you need to stop eating so much chocolate. As if that was it, that I sat there at home eating chocolate all the time.

"I had postnatal depression at the time as well, and most did not care. They didn't care about the postnatal depression, they didn't care about the hyperemesis, they didn't care about the thyroid problem, but they would talk about the weight all the time. It was like that was the part that was the most important thing apparently. Now I have finally got my thyroid under control I've lost weight again and get so many reactions that I look slimmer, as if that's the most important thing. I often point out that, no, I look healthier or fitter because my body is functioning as it should and that's what's actually important.

"And there's so much evidence that, for women of reproductive age, having a BMI of about 27, 28 is actually pretty healthy. If you actually look at a lot of the outcomes. It was the same with Covid. If you broke down that Covid and weight data, actually there was a lot of evidence to show that it was one of the lowest risk categories. Yet still this concept of, oh no, you haven't got the exact perfect BMI. And the whole thing around breastfeeding being good for weight

loss, and losing calories and don't eat more, and why are we not teaching women to fuel their bodies, to eat for nutrition? Don't starve yourself, you're growing a baby, you're breastfeeding a baby … why isn't that the emphasis?" (Amy Brown)

As can be seen from Amy's story, the focus on using BMI as a single measure of health can potentially affect all women. This emphasis is causing harm to women, it's leading some professionals and birth workers to focus on the wrong things, and there's no evidence that it's leading to improvements.

A different perspective

There is some positive news. A growing body of evidence and thinking is challenging the myths and opinions that make up our current approach. Many people are highlighting the problems and providing a more person-centred perspective. It's increasingly clear that a BMI-focused approach isn't evidence-based, respectful, proportional, or logical. When we examine the issues and the evidence relating to the individual tests, interventions and restrictions that are offered, as I will do in the next few chapters, it turns out that there is a bigger picture. There is also some evidence that you can increase your chances of a good outcome not by following the BMI-focused, opinion-based obstetric guidelines, but by seeking a caregiver who can offer individualised care and a setting and situation that will support your body to birth optimally.

Let's look at the evidence.

4. Pregnancy outcomes and evidence

One of the key tenets of the BMI-focused approach taken within the maternity services is the claim that women who have a higher BMI are at increased risk of experiencing a number of unwanted or adverse outcomes. The scariest-sounding one is stillbirth. A worrying number of larger women have told myself and other researchers that stillbirth risk has been used to get them to agree to additional tests and interventions, including ultrasound scans, induction of labour, and giving birth in a consultant unit instead of at home or in a midwifery-led unit. Often, the stillbirth risk is emphasised after the woman declines a test or intervention, or expresses a desire for something seen as 'alternative'.

Other risks that larger women are told about include pre-eclampsia, gestational diabetes, having a large baby (macrosomia), and having a higher chance of a caesarean section. But, as I explained in the previous chapter, the evidence underpinning these claims isn't always robust. So in this chapter I'm going to look at the data relating to the outcomes that we are told that women with a higher BMI are at higher risk of experiencing. That's the first step towards deciding whether or not you want to accept the tests, interventions, and restrictions that are being offered in the hope of reducing your chance of experiencing certain things.

In fact, when we look at the evidence relating to higher BMI and birth outcomes rather than relying on the opinion of those who wrote the guidelines, there are three bits of good news. If you are healthy, your BMI has little impact on pregnancy and birth outcomes. The chance of experiencing unwanted outcomes is lower than you might have been led to believe. And there are decisions that you can make which will further increase your chance of having a straightforward birth, and reduce the chance of you or your baby experiencing problems. In this and the next three chapters, I'll explain the evidence behind these three statements in detail.

The good news about pregnancy, BMI and risk

In 2014, a paper from an important research study caused a bit of a stir when it showed that some of the beliefs that people held about pregnancy, BMI, and risk weren't actually true. A research project called the Birthplace in England study was being carried out by the National Perinatal Epidemiology Unit at Oxford University, England. The researchers were looking at outcomes and interventions in relation to planned place of birth, and they had gathered data from tens of thousands of women and babies. Several important papers emerged from this study, and one of them looked specifically at the outcomes of 17,230 women who had a BMI of 35 kg/m^2 or more but no other risk factors.

This particular study wasn't comparing place of birth, though. The women had followed the standard advice given to those with a BMI of 35 kg/m^2 or more, which was to give birth in an obstetric unit. But, as the researchers pointed out, the advice to birth in hospital is *"based on consensus rather than high quality evidence"* (Hollowell *et al* 2014).

Their findings confirmed some important things. The first was that only 12.9% of the women who had a higher BMI also had a pre-existing medical condition or risk factor (such as diabetes or asthma) at the onset of pregnancy. By 37 weeks of pregnancy, 45.4% of the women had either a pre-existing or new risk factor or medical condition (such as pre-eclampsia), but more than half of those with a higher BMI had no risk factors at all (Hollowell *et al* 2014).

Some people had long been saying how important it is that we distinguish between women who have a higher BMI but are healthy, and women who have a higher BMI and who also have one or more health conditions which may lead to poorer outcomes if we don't offer appropriate care, tests, and/or interventions. Hollowell *et al*'s (2014) study helped show that there are more women in the first group (healthy and higher BMI) than most people think.

The findings of this study did show that, where women

were otherwise healthy and simply had a higher BMI but no other risk factors, they were a bit more likely to experience certain outcomes than women of 'normal weight'. These things included being told that they needed to have their labour augmented (speeded up) with an oxytocin drip, and/or that they needed a caesarean. But the difference in the rate of adverse outcomes between the two groups of women was modest (Hollowell *et al* 2014). More modest than lots of people had previously thought, especially for women who were giving birth to a second or later baby. And, as I will also discuss below, this might be more about caregivers and guidelines than BMI.

In the same year, a Dutch study of midwife-led practices also confirmed that women who were healthy and had a higher BMI were no more likely to be referred to obstetric care than women of 'normal weight' (Daemers *et al* 2014). The research team found that 55% of those women remained in midwifery-led care throughout pregnancy, and 30% of them gave birth in midwifery-led settings. Again, those who had given birth before had an even higher chance of avoiding complications.

In Daemers *et al*'s (2014) research, the only significant difference in outcomes was that 3.3% of healthy women with a higher BMI who remained in midwife-led care gave birth to a large for gestational age (LGA) baby compared to 1.9% of women of 'normal weight'. I'll look at the evidence relating to large babies later in this chapter, but that isn't a significant difference when we consider the absolute numbers.

Researchers also looked at how many women who have a higher BMI have a healthy pregnancy (Relph *et al* 2021). Their findings are similar to those above. They found that more than half of the women who had no pre-existing medical or early obstetric complications but who were told they were 'at risk' because of having a higher BMI went on to have a healthy, uncomplicated pregnancy (Relph *et al* 2021).

In fact, all of these research studies show the same things. Having a higher BMI does not mean that complications are inevitable. If you are healthy, BMI has little impact on pregnancy and birth outcomes. In fact, we need to question whether BMI is even an independent risk factor for an adverse outcome. It's true, as I'll detail below, that people with a higher BMI have a greater chance of experiencing some health conditions. But the difference often isn't that great, the conditions are experienced by people with a lower BMI as well, and plenty of people with a higher BMI don't develop them. All of which implies that we should be focusing on spotting the conditions rather than on someone's BMI. Given the evidence, it is inappropriate to consider high BMI as a risk factor in the same way that we see things like high blood pressure or heart disease as risk factors.

If you have midwifery-led care or give birth in a midwifery-led setting, you have an even better chance of a straightforward vaginal birth and a lower chance of some adverse outcomes. But many women who have a higher BMI have a healthy pregnancy and a straightforward birth even if they give birth in hospital, where obstetric intervention is more likely. The findings on place of birth highlight that it is inappropriate to deny women with a higher BMI the chance to give birth in midwifery-led settings, as some of the researchers point out: *"Care in lower-risk settings can be considered as their outcomes appear similar to those reported for low-risk nulliparous women."* (Relph *et al* 2021)

In 2018, another important paper on the setting of care was published in the UK, and it made things even clearer for those who were concerned about the treatment of plus size women. It's known as the UKMidSS study, which stands for the UK Midwifery Study System. UKMidSS is a national data collection platform used to gather information about women who give birth and babies who are born in a midwifery-led unit (MLU) in the UK. These anonymously gathered data can be used by researchers to look at the outcomes of midwifery-led care in these units.

This 2018 study by Rowe *et al* looked at women with a BMI of 35 kg/m^2 or higher who were admitted to alongside MLUs in the UK. These are units that are in or next to a hospital but where care is given by midwives. They are sometimes called birth centres, and the environment is often more relaxed than in an obstetric unit.

Rowe *et al* (2018) analysed data from 1122 women with a BMI of 35 kg/m^2 or more, and compared their outcomes with data from 1949 comparison women, who had a BMI of less than 35 kg/m^2. The researchers used something called a composite outcome to see if there was a difference in outcomes between women in different BMI categories. This involves looking at several different unwanted outcomes at the same time, and it can help show differences even when the absolute chance of a particular poor outcome is low. The outcomes included augmentation (acceleration of labour), instrumental birth, caesarean, maternal blood transfusion, a severe (third or fourth degree) tear, or the woman needing to be moved to higher level care. Rowe *et al* (2018) found that women with a BMI of 35 kg/m^2 or more were no more likely to experience this composite outcome than women with a 'normal' BMI.

Something very interesting appears when we look at the straightforward vaginal birth rate in different BMI categories. In Rowe *et al*'s study, 96.3% of women who had a BMI of 35 kg/m^2 and were having a second or later baby in a MLU had a straightforward vaginal birth. This is actually higher than the 93.5% of women with a 'normal' BMI who had a straightforward vaginal birth. It's important to acknowledge that women who opt for care in an MLU are self-selected, so they may be more motivated to do things to increase their chances of having this outcome. But if you are reading this as someone with a higher BMI and considering your options, that's not bad news at all. It confirms the value and importance of carefully considering the kind of care that will help you have the birth you want.

The chance of having a straightforward vaginal birth is a bit lower for women having their first baby, but the data again show that this isn't really about BMI. The women who had a

BMI of 35 kg/m^2 or more and were having their first baby had a 67.9% chance of having a straightforward vaginal birth, compared to 69.8% of those who were similar except for having a 'normal' BMI (Rowe *et al* 2018). Caesarean rates were also low and similar.

These studies confirm what I wrote above about it being important to differentiate between being healthy and having a higher BMI. The two are not linked in the way that some people want us to believe that they are. Healthy plus size women have a higher chance of having a straightforward birth with good outcomes than they do of having a problem. We can see that there is often very little or no difference in outcomes between women who have a higher BMI and women with a BMI that is considered 'normal'. Sometimes, larger women have an advantage. We also know from the data that women who have given birth before have a lower chance of problems. But that doesn't mean it's bad news for those who are having their first baby. Because, as all of these studies show, the chance of a problem is much lower than we are often told and opting for midwifery-led care and/or a midwifery-led setting for labour and birth gives you (and, in fact, all women, regardless of BMI) a higher chance of avoiding unnecessary interventions and unwanted outcomes.

Back to absolute and relative risk

I have already mentioned the idea of absolute and relative risk, and that it's important to understand the difference. This is a key element in the point I made above about how, even when people with a higher BMI do have a higher chance of experiencing certain things, the difference or the risk isn't always as significant as might be implied.

This point was made by Amy Brown (2019) in her book, *Informed is Best*. She looked at some of the studies which show that higher BMI is linked with an increased chance of certain birth outcomes, and then unpacked the data to show how, when we look at absolute risk, the picture looks different.

"[Cedergren *et al* 2004] *looked at birth outcomes for 805,275 pregnant women in Sweden according to their weight. They compared outcomes for women who were a healthy BMI (19-26) to those with a BMI of 29-35 (obese), 35-40 (morbidly obese) and more than 40 (very morbidly obese). I'm not sure what happened to the women who would have been considered overweight (BMI 27-28).*

"In the abstract the authors focus on comparing women with a BMI over 40 and those with a healthy BMI, using relative risk to state that those with a BMI over 40 were:

- *4.8 times more likely to have pre-eclampsia*
- *2.8 times more likely to have a stillbirth*
- *2.7 times more likely to have a c-section*
- *3.4 times more likely to have a neonatal death*

"The abstract does sound scary. 'Maternal morbid obesity in early pregnancy is strongly associated with a number of pregnancy complications and perinatal conditions.' However, when you look at the individual absolute risk *for women with a healthy BMI compared to a BMI over 40 they showed risks of:*

- *1.4% versus 3.5% for pre-eclampsia*
- *0.3% versus 0.8% for a stillbirth*
- *10.9% versus 34% for a caesarean section*
- *0.1% versus 0.4% for neonatal death."* (Brown 2019: 328)

Brown (2019) also looked at the findings of a Canadian study (Schummers *et al* 2015), which included a wider range of participants with more varied racial backgrounds. The results were similar. That is, the chance of having an adverse outcome does rise to some extent as BMI increases, but the absolute chance of an adverse outcome remains low. Many women find absolute risk far more helpful as a basis for making decisions about their care. I'll come back to the discussion about stillbirth at the end of this chapter.

Brown (2019) also points out that researchers compared the two extremes of the data when they calculated relative risk. In other words, they took the group with the highest chance of a problem and compared their risk to the group with the lowest chance of a problem. As the chance of an unwanted outcome often increases only slightly with each BMI category, the risk for someone with a BMI of 31 kg/m^2 may be barely (if any) higher than the risk for someone with a BMI of 26 kg/m^2. Comparing the very lowest and the very highest risk figure masks that nuance, and is only accurate for the 5% of women in the UK (or 1 in 20) who have a BMI over 40 kg/m^2. This doesn't mean that intervention is warranted for those with a very high BMI either, by the way. There is also a much bigger picture, as Brown explains:

"What's important is that although the individual risk does increase as BMI increases a) those with a healthy BMI can still have the complication and b) it is a small overall risk, not a definitive. The only one that particularly stands out is the c-section rate, but flip that on its head: two thirds of women with a BMI over 40 still give birth without a c-section" (Brown 2019: 328-29).

Actually, there is even more that we can say about why plus size women are more likely to have a caesarean, so let's look at that next, because it illustrates another really important point about risk and outcomes.

The chance of having a caesarean

We saw from the data analysed by Brown (2019) that the most likely unwanted outcome experienced by women with a higher BMI is to have a caesarean birth. I realise that some women want and request a caesarean, but I have written unwanted in the previous sentence because most do not. A caesarean has a number of risks compared to a physiological, vaginal birth (Sandall *et al* 2018), so many people feel it is better to have one only if medically necessary.

A large number of studies from around the world over many years show that women with a higher BMI are far more likely to end up with a caesarean than those with a lower BMI (Poobalan *et al* 2009, Kominiarek *et al* 2010, Hollowell *et al*

2014, Declerq *et al* 2015, Ellekjaer *et al* 2017, Pettersen-Dahl *et al* 2018, Vats *et al* 2021, Panda *et al* 2022, Eloranta *et al* 2023).

There is an important difference between the outcome of a caesarean and some of the other unwanted outcomes that I mentioned above, however. A caesarean doesn't just happen as a 'natural' outcome of pregnancy. It is the result of one or more people making a decision, and then taking action. Usually, a clinician will recommend a caesarean, the woman decides whether to accept or decline the offer and, if she agrees to have a caesarean, a number of people work together in a specialised way to make this happen. This makes it a very different kind of outcome from stillbirth, or pre-eclampsia. Yes, those outcomes can be affected by someone's decisions, and there is often room for debate on how conditions are defined and categorised, but caesareans can only ever happen when people make them happen.

It's important to bear this in mind because, as I discussed in earlier chapters, people with a higher BMI receive less support and experience more stigma. We know some people think that larger women are less able to give birth vaginally (more on this in chapter six), and we know that weight bias exists but isn't taken into account in maternity care guidelines (Nagpal *et al* 2022). We also have clear evidence showing that *"decisions to perform a* [caesarean] *are, on occasion, based on clinicians' personal beliefs and interpretation."* (Panda *et al* 2022).

While some clinicians will tell you that women with a higher BMI are more likely to have a caesarean because of reasons to do with their weight or size, we have to consider the possibility that the increased chance of being told you need a caesarean if you have a higher BMI may be wholly or partly because of the beliefs and attitudes held by health professionals, and by the way they and others treat you during your pregnancy and birth. Declerq *et al* (2015) discussed in their analysis how this happens in the USA, where women with a high BMI are far more likely than women with a lower BMI to be told they need a caesarean, even if they are healthy and have no other risk factors.

I want to return to the UKMidSS study that I discussed above (Rowe *et al* 2018). While the women in this study (which looked at outcomes in midwifery-led units) showed that women with a BMI of 35 kg/m^2 or more were more likely to have an in-labour caesarean than women with a 'normal' BMI, caesarean rates were low in both groups, and the absolute difference was small. Rowe *et al* (2018) found that 4.7% of women with a BMI of 35 kg/m^2 or more had a caesarean, compared to 4.1% of women who had a BMI in the 'normal' range. This is barely different at all.

Again, it may also be that the risk labelling that is applied to plus sized women means that they are more likely to end up with interventions that increase the chance of a caesarean. We call this kind of risk an iatrogenic risk, and this just means that a complication, disease, or adverse outcome (in this case caesarean) is caused by medical activity, which might be an intervention, error, attitude, or inappropriate diagnosis. I will look at how this happens in labour and birth in chapter six.

As you've now seen, your chance of being told you need intervention differs according to the type of care you receive, where you give birth, and what kind of caregiver you have. This doesn't just apply to plus size women. We have lots of data showing that women and babies have better outcomes and fewer interventions when they have midwife-led care. Sandall *et al* (2016) undertook a review of 15 trials involving 17,674 women and found that *"women who received midwife-led continuity models of care were less likely to experience intervention and more likely to be satisfied with their care with at least comparable adverse outcomes for women or their infants than women who received other models of care."*

Lots of data also show that women who plan home birth have a higher chance of experiencing straightforward vaginal birth and less chance of having certain unwanted outcomes, including severe perineal trauma or haemorrhage (Scarf *et al* 2018, Olsen & Clausen 2023). It is also clear that home birth is just as safe as hospital birth for healthy women (Scarf *et al* 2018, Hutton *et al* 2019). In fact, it's very clear that the type of care that women receive makes a difference in several ways. This may sound like bad news, and it's certainly not ideal if we focus on the so-called 'postcode lottery' element of modern health care. But knowing that the environment of care and the people who are around you can affect outcomes is actually one of the most important things that you can learn about if you have a higher BMI. This knowledge is the starting point for getting more informed and taking control of your decisions, which will improve your chance of getting the care and the outcomes you need and want.

The risks of higher BMI: looking at the numbers

I have mentioned that the claims made within guidelines about higher BMI women being at much greater risk of certain outcomes don't always stand up to scrutiny. I also explained that, even when there is a slight increase in the chance of complications for those with a very high BMI at a population level, there is often only a tiny increased chance on an individual level. It's time I provided the evidence for you to examine for yourself.

There are a few situations that can arise in pregnancy that the writers of obstetric guidelines are particularly concerned about when it comes to plus size women. These include pre-eclampsia and hypertension, gestational diabetes, whether a baby is especially big, thromboembolism, and then a number of outcomes that may affect babies. Let's look at each of those in turn.

Pre-eclampsia

Pre-eclampsia is a condition that can develop during pregnancy, usually after about 20 weeks. Early signs of pre-eclampsia include hypertension (high blood pressure) and proteinuria (protein in your urine). Other symptoms such as oedema (swelling), headache and visual disturbance can develop in later stages of the condition.

Not all women who develop hypertension or pre-eclampsia will have serious problems. But pre-eclampsia can become serious if not appropriately diagnosed and managed. This is why antenatal check-ups include tests to help identify early signs, such as blood pressure checks, urine analysis, and being asked to report any oedema (swelling), headaches or visual disturbances. Most women with pre-eclampsia will be successfully treated with medication. Some will be offered induction. Pre-eclampsia resolves once a baby is born.

Globally, pre-eclampsia affects about 1 in 20 pregnancies (Abalos *et al* 2013, RCOG 2022). It is more likely to occur in women who already have high blood pressure or certain medical conditions (including kidney disease and type 1 and type 2 diabetes), who are pregnant for the first time, who have a multiple pregnancy, or who are older.

Several studies have shown that women who have a high BMI are more likely to develop pre-eclampsia than women with a lower BMI, and the chance of pre-eclampsia increases as BMI increases (O'Brien *et al* 2003, Cedergren *et al* 2004, Cnossen et al 2007, Wang *et al* 2013, Schummers *et al* 2015, Poorolajal & Jenabi 2016, Bartsch *et al* 2016, Townsend *et al* 2019). Not all of these studies break the risk down by BMI category, but Schummers *et al* (2015) have done this, and their data showed that the chance of developing pre-eclampsia by BMI category was:

2.4% (1 in 40) of women with BMI less than 18.5 kg/m^2
3.4% (1 in 29) of women with BMI of 18.5-<25 kg/m^2
6.4% (1 in 16) of women with BMI of 25-<30 kg/m^2
10% (1 in 10) of women with BMI of 30-<35 kg/m^2
12.8% (1 in 8) of women with BMI of 35-<40 kg/m.
16.3% (1 in 6) of women with BMI of 40 kg/m^2 or more.

I think it can also help to turn these figures around. Nearly 84% of women in the highest BMI category do not experience pre-eclampsia. Pre-eclampsia can be managed. Drugs can lower blood pressure, and in severe cases a woman may be offered an induction or caesarean to deliver the baby early. Women with a higher BMI are often offered aspirin to prevent pre-eclampsia, which I discuss in chapter five.

Gestational diabetes

The term diabetes is used to describe a condition in which someone isn't producing enough insulin to regulate the amount of glucose (sugar) in their blood. There are several different forms of diabetes, as I described in chapter two. As a reminder, type 1 diabetes is a lifelong condition in which someone can't produce enough insulin in their body. Type 2 diabetes is the kind that people may develop as they get older (although it's possible for children to develop it too), in which they either aren't producing enough insulin or their body has become resistant to insulin. Gestational diabetes mellitus (GDM) is a condition caused by pregnancy hormones, which can create insulin resistance in the mother. The hormones that lead to a diagnosis of gestational diabetes will resolve once the placenta is out. When diabetes is found in pregnancy, it may be type 2 diabetes, which won't disappear after birth.

Women with a higher BMI have a greater chance of being diagnosed with gestational diabetes than women with a lower BMI. Just as with pre-eclampsia, the chance of being diagnosed with gestational diabetes increases in each BMI category, but the absolute figures (which vary according to the data used to calculate them and the screening test used) are not as high as some people think.

Overall, about 4-5% of pregnant women are diagnosed with gestational diabetes in the UK (RCOG 2021), which is one in every 20. It is more common in those with a family history of GDM, in those of South Asian, Chinese, African-Caribbean or Middle Eastern descent, and in women who have a higher BMI (RCOG 2021). The paper cited in the RCOG guidance (Denison *et al* 2018) is an older study by Weiss *et al* (2004). They showed that GDM was diagnosed in:

2.3% of women (1 in 42) with a BMI of less than 30 kg/m^2
6.3% of women (1 in 16) with a BMI of 30-34.9 kg/m^2
9.5% of women (1 in 10) with a BMI of 35 kg/m^2 or higher

More recent data show that the chance of being diagnosed as having gestational diabetes is higher in all BMI categories than in the Weiss *et al* (2004) study. For instance, Martin *et al* (2015) looked at Australian data and found GDM rates to be:

6.74% of women with a BMI of 25-29.9 kg/m^2
13.42% of women with a BMI of 30-34.9 kg/m^2
12.79% of women with a BMI of 35-39.9 kg/m^2
20.00% of women with a BMI of 40 kg/m^2 or higher

In Canada, Schummers *et al* (2015) found GDM rates to be:

5.4% of women with a BMI of less than 18.5 kg/m^2
6.1% of women with a BMI of 18.5-<25 kg/m^2
9.7% of women with a BMI of 25-<30 kg/m^2
13.7% of women with a BMI of 30-<35 kg/m^2
16.6% of women with a BMI of 35-<40 kg/m^2
20.8% of women with a BMI of 40 kg/m^2 or higher

The differences in these findings illustrate one of the most frustrating aspects of the evidence. The data on the chance of being diagnosed with GDM vary because the cut-off points and definitions of GDM vary, both over time and by place. Many people have voiced frustration at these changing criteria. Shipton *et al* (2022) show that, *"In Australia, diagnostic criteria changes increased GDM diagnoses by 35%, without detectable population-level improvement in most perinatal outcomes."* The same authors also pointed out that almost no attention has been paid to what women think and feel about gestational diabetes screening and treatment.

No matter which study and cut-off points we look at, the majority of larger women don't develop gestational diabetes. More on GDM screening and treatment in chapter five.

Large babies and shoulder dystocia

Another concern is about whether women with a higher BMI will have a larger baby. The medical term for a large baby is macrosomia, and most health care systems deem a baby to be large when they weigh 4kg (8lbs 13oz) or more.

Most babies who are large do not have any problems, but a few will experience problems when being born, including shoulder dystocia, where their shoulders get stuck and may need help to be born. More on this in chapter five. Women who are thought to have a larger baby are more at risk of being told they need induction or caesarean, and may be more likely to have a tear, although all of these things are affected by several other factors as well (Beta *et al* 2019).

Larger babies sometimes experience problems after birth, although this may be more about whether diabetes (which can also lead to babies being larger, especially if it is poorly controlled) is an issue rather than anything to do with their size *per se*. This is another example of where it may be more important to consider a woman's metabolic health rather than use her BMI or weight as a proxy for health.

A number of studies show that women with a higher BMI have a higher chance of having a large baby than women with a lower BMI (Sebire *et al* 2001, Cedergren *et al* 2004, Bhattacharya *et al* 2007, Gaudet *et al* 2014). But, just as with the other conditions we have looked at, the issues are complex. The increased chance of having a larger baby isn't as high as some people think. Some studies (Sebire *et al* 2001, Cedergren *et al* 2004) only give data on relative risk, which means it's not possible to calculate the actual chance that women in particular BMI categories will have a larger baby. The majority of women who have a higher BMI do not have a large baby, and plenty of those who have a lower BMI do have large babies. Most large babies are fine, and there are downsides to the screening and prevention strategies that are offered in this area, which I will discuss in chapters five and six. For example, the evidence doesn't support offering induction for a suspected large baby (Wickham 2021a).

There are different ways of defining a large baby in medical circles. One is to estimate or measure the size of the baby relative to what we would expect the average baby to weigh at a particular stage of pregnancy. These averages are used to create growth charts, and the combination of ways of measuring babies' sizes (which include midwives' or doctors' hands, tape measures or ultrasound scans) and mapping them onto growth charts is what leads us to say that some babies are 'small for gestational age' (SGA) or 'large for gestational age' (LGA). A large for gestational age baby is one whose estimated or actual birth weight is equal to or greater than the weight which marks the 90th (or sometimes the 95th) percentile for their gestational age on whatever growth chart is being used locally. This just means that a baby is (or is estimated to be) in the top ten (or five) per cent of babies by their weight at that particular stage of pregnancy. A small for gestational age baby is one whose estimated or actual weight is below the tenth or fifth centile. Again, this varies around the world. So this is a more relative (to other babies) measurement, whereas an actual weight (such as 4kg) is a more absolute measurement, as the same cut-off point is used for every baby. I will discuss ultrasound scans in chapter five.

One of the reviews which gives us data on both LGA and macrosomia rates is that by Gaudet *et al* (2014), who analysed data from high- and middle-income countries. They showed that women with a BMI of 30 kg/m^2 or above were more likely than women with a 'normal' BMI to have a larger baby. Their results suggest that about one in six of the women in the included studies whose BMI was 'average' or 'underweight' gave birth to an LGA baby, and about one in five of the women in these studies who had a BMI of 30 kg/m^2 gave birth to an LGA baby.

A closer look at the data in the Gaudet *et al* (2014) study gives a clue as to why the rate of LGA babies is higher in both groups than is often seen in practice. Several of the included studies were focused on women who had diabetes or gestational diabetes, who we know have a higher chance of having a larger baby. So yes, the results can tell us about the relative chance of having a larger baby in that particular data set, but they can also make it appear that the chance of having a larger baby is higher across the board than it really is. I am including these data because they show that, for those women who do have gestational diabetes or are in a 'higher risk' category (for reasons other than their BMI), there is still a very good chance of having a baby who is not large for gestational age. But I have included this explanation as a reminder of why it is important to look more deeply at the research, rather than relying on advice from those who do not have the ability, time, or inclination to dig into the data.

You may recall that I looked at a study by Daemers *et al* (2014) earlier in this chapter. I want to remind you of their finding that 3.3% of healthy women with a higher BMI gave birth to a large for gestational age baby compared to 1.9% of women of 'normal weight.' Again, it is important that we look at whether someone is healthy or has actual medical conditions rather than just at what their BMI is.

I also want to reiterate the point that that being on one or other end of the size spectrum doesn't mean anything in itself. This is especially true when a baby is estimated to be large. It may be that your baby is simply a future rugby player in the making. Perhaps both parents are over six foot, or your family just tend to grow large babies. Yes, some babies are genuinely, unexpectedly, and problematically large. But some are simply constitutionally large. When we carry out an individualised assessment of a family, there is sometimes good reason that a baby is nearer to one or other end of the spectrum. Just as with BMI, physical measurement is a crude tool by which to assess health, risk, and wellbeing.

I mentioned at the beginning of this section that one of the concerns about large babies is that they are more likely to experience shoulder dystocia, so I want to add some data on this too. Most large babies don't experience shoulder dystocia (Gross *et al* 1987, RCOG 2012). In fact 94% of babies over 4kg in Beta *et al*'s (2019) study did not have shoulder dystocia. When it does happen, midwives and doctors are trained to respond and it only very rarely has serious consequences.

Hollowell *et al* (2014) looked at labour and birth outcomes according to maternal BMI and did not find higher BMI to be an independent risk factor for shoulder dystocia. In fact, no study has ever accurately predicted which babies will have shoulder dystocia (Leung *et al* 2011, RCOG 2012, Boulvain *et al* 2016). Neither has any study predicted which babies will experience negative effects as a result of experiencing shoulder dystocia (RCOG 2012, Boulvain *et al* 2016, Wickham 2021a). I will return to the screening and treatment measures related to predicting macrosomia in chapters five and six.

Venous thromboembolism

Thromboembolism is the medical term for what happens when a blood clot (or thrombus) forms in a blood vessel and is then carried through the blood until it blocks another blood vessel (with the blockage being called an embolus). The word embolus describes the state of being blocked and while both arteries and veins can be affected by thromboembolism, it is venous (vein) thromboembolisms that are of more concern in pregnancy. This condition isn't common but can be serious. It can cause organ damage and may be fatal if left untreated.

Venous thromboembolism is often abbreviated as VTE. It can occur in a number of forms, and the two that we are most concerned about in pregnancy are known as deep vein thrombosis (DVT) and pulmonary embolism (PE).

DVTs are otherwise known as a blood clot in the leg. DVTs are most commonly seen in the calves, but they may appear elsewhere. Symptoms can include swelling, throbbing, red or darkened skin, warmth, pain, and cramps in just one leg. You may or may not see a hardened vein. You do not have to have all of the symptoms to have a DVT. If you think you may have a DVT, seek medical help immediately.

A PE is a blood clot that has lodged in the lung. Symptoms

of a PE include having sudden shortness of breath, very fast breathing, or chest pain. Someone with a PE may cough up some blood, and their lips or fingers may change colour as there is less oxygen in their blood. The skin of a white person who has less circulating oxygen can appear to be blue (cyanosis). In people with black or brown skin, a lack of oxygen can appear as more of a grey or white colour, while the area around the eyes can seem grey or blue. This is very rare but a life-threatening condition for which you should seek immediate, emergency medical help.

A number of factors can increase someone's chance of developing a VTE. One of them is pregnancy, and other risk factors for VTE include having a higher BMI (whether or not you're pregnant), being older, having a family history of this condition, having certain chronic diseases (such as heart or lung disease), and sitting or lying still for a long time. This last factor can include being in bed after surgery or, as people are aware these days, sitting still on a long-haul flight. The foot twirling and leg exercises on the safety information card in your seat pocket are designed to help reduce the risk of DVT by improving your circulation.

VTE is something that all midwives and doctors are urged to be aware of and focus on (RCOG 2015). The research that is carried out in the UK into the rare but awful situation where mothers die during and just after pregnancy (Knight *et al* 2022) shows that VTE is the leading medical or direct cause of maternal deaths in pregnancy and up until six weeks after the baby is born. VTE is also one of the leading causes of maternal deaths in the USA (Creanga *et al* 2017) and Australia (Australian Institute of Health and Welfare 2022b). The researchers suggested that, *"...several of these deaths could be prevented with improvements to care."* (Knight *et al* 2022). This is why the identification of those at risk of VTE and the offering of preventative measures for some women has become a key focus of guidelines (Denison *et al* 2018, ACOG 2021, RANZCOG 2022).

But the question of which women should be offered

preventative measures is a contentious one. This is another situation in which lots of women will be told they have risk factors and offered preventative medication for a very serious condition that would only be experienced by very few people. Some women find this really frustrating as the medication offered to prevent VTE potentially has more unwanted effects than foot twirling, but I'll come back to that.

First, let's look at the data from a study of almost two and a half million women who gave birth in California between 2008 and 2012. This is the largest study I could find, and in this case size matters very much, because VTE is less common than the other conditions I've discussed. So we need lots of data in order to get an accurate picture of how often it occurs.

The researchers share separate figures for the chance of experiencing VTE during pregnancy and the chance of experiencing this after the birth. That's because the chance is higher for *all* women in the postnatal period.

Butwick *et al* (2019) looked at actual cases of VTE and showed that, during pregnancy, VTE was experienced by:

2.3 in 10,000 (1 in 4348) women with BMI up to 18.4 kg/m^2.
3.0 in 10,000 (1 in 3333) women with BMI of 18.5-24.9 kg/m^2.
3.8 in 10,000 (1 in 2632) women with BMI of 25-29.9 kg/m^2.
4.2 in 10,000 (1 in 2380) women with BMI of 30-34.9 kg/m^2.
4.7 in 10,000 (1 in 2128) women with BMI of 35-39.9 kg/m^2.
10.6 in 10,000 (1 in 943) women with BMI 40 kg/m^2 or more.

In the postnatal period, VTE was experienced by:

2.0 in 10,000 (1 in 5000) women with BMI up to 18.4 kg/m^2.
3.1 in 10,000 (1 in 3226) women with BMI of 18.5-24.9 kg/m^2.
3.9 in 10,000 (1 in 2564) women with BMI of 25-29.9 kg/m^2.
5.6 in 10,000 (1 in 1786) women with BMI of 30-34.9 kg/m^2.
9.0 in 10,000 (1 in 1111) women with BMI of 35-39.9 kg/m^2.
13.2 in 10,000 (1 in 758) women with BMI 40 kg/m^2 or more.

Nowadays, in some countries, women believed to have an increased chance of VTE are offered a preventative medicine called low molecular weight heparin (LMWH). Women with a higher BMI are among those who are offered heparin injections. This treatment is controversial, and in fact most countries don't offer it during pregnancy, which means that the researchers questioning it have tended to focus their papers on whether or not it is beneficial after birth. So please see the sections on heparin and preventing venous thromboembolism in chapters five and seven, where I discuss the pros and cons of these injections and the conversations that are happening in this area.

BMI and other outcomes for babies

I already mentioned some of the statistics on BMI and stillbirth when I wrote about absolute and relative risk earlier in this chapter, and I've also discussed macrosomia. But it's important to look more closely at a few other fetal and neonatal outcomes.

Guidelines in many high-income countries relating to BMI often state that stillbirth, preterm birth, congenital abnormalities, and neonatal death are also increased when women have a higher BMI (Denison *et al* 2018, ACOG 2021, RANZCOG 2022). It is true that some studies do show that some of these things occur more often in women who have a higher BMI. But we often have no idea why this is the case (Woolner & Bhattacharya 2015). When you dig into the research studies and also look at the wider issues, it turns out that the relationship between BMI and outcomes for babies isn't always negative.

Preterm birth

Preterm birth is a good example of how issues relating to BMI and birth outcomes aren't straightforward. Some studies have found that the chance of preterm birth increases with higher BMI (Liu *et al* 2019, Slack *et al* 2019). But a much larger number of studies have shown the opposite: that women with a higher pre-pregnancy BMI are less likely to have a preterm baby than women with a lower BMI (Schieve *et al* 2000, Sebire *et al* 2001, Kumari 2001, Hendler *et al* 2005, Goldenberg *et al* 2008, Kashanian *et al* 2019, Calix *et al* 2020, Baer *et al* 2022). For example, Baer *et al* (2022) found that *"women with BMI ≥30.0 kg/m² were at decreased risk of a spontaneous preterm birth with intact membranes between 32 and 36 weeks."*

This is another example of the so-called obesity paradox, where having a higher BMI may actually be an advantage. But it's hard to put numbers to this. That's because, as Kurz and König (2020) explain in their analysis of association between higher BMI and preterm birth, the studies tend to be observational. I'm not going to disparage observational studies because, in situations where there aren't good trial data, or where trials aren't the best way of finding out the answer to something, their findings can be very useful. But all types of studies have limitations, and it's important to be careful about what conclusions we draw from them.

For example, Kurz & König (2020) discussed the cohort study by Liu *et al* (2019) *"which reported a statistically significant association between pre-pregnancy obesity and increased risk of preterm birth."* They explained how the kind of data they looked at aren't enough to help us know if one thing (BMI) causes another (preterm birth). One reason for this is that several of the conditions that I have discussed in this chapter are inter-related and it can be hard to separate out different factors in order to see what's going on. We've already discussed pre-eclampsia, which we know occurs more frequently in women with a higher BMI, and pre-eclampsia is also associated with preterm birth (RCOG 2022). But when studies look at women who have a higher BMI and who don't develop conditions like pre-eclampsia, that's when we see that higher BMI is protective against preterm birth.

We still have a lot to learn. As Kurz and König (2020)

pointed out, we know that preterm birth is partly influenced by genetics, we know that BMI is influenced by genetics, and we know that mothers and their babies share some genes. Is it possible that someone's genetic make-up is influencing both their BMI *and* their chance of having a preterm baby? We just don't know. Frustratingly, far more research funding is put towards studies which align with the status quo and our culture's existing values and assumptions than towards areas where findings show something different or challenge the dominant rationality. In a sense, this is inevitable, because funding often derives from pharmaceutical and technology companies. It's important to remain aware of the economic issues that relate to knowledge, research and evidence, as there is an inbuilt bias towards researching the use of tests and interventions which can be developed for profit.

Congenital abnormalities

When we look at the question of congenital abnormalities in babies born to women with a higher BMI, the complexity of underlying factors and the assumptions that our culture makes about the effect of size and weight make this another tricky area to examine.

Congenital abnormalities (which refers to abnormalities that a baby is born with) result from genetic, environmental, nutritional, and/or infectious factors. These are all factors that are also known to have a potential impact on someone's size and BMI. So it may be that one of these factors leads to or is associated with higher BMI *and* a greater chance of congenital abnormalities, rather than higher BMI being the cause of a congenital abnormality in itself.

Some studies show that congenital abnormalities are seen more often in babies born to women with a high BMI, and that the risk increases with each BMI category (Pressman & Običan 2023). This may prove to be the case, but the relationships are complex, the studies aren't always as robust as we might like, and we haven't properly unpacked the wider issues and factors that influence BMI. Ironically, dieting may itself be part of the problem, as some plus size women may have been restricting their nutrient intake. But we don't have the right research to know whether this is or isn't the case.

Factors relating to the difficulty of collecting data on rare but important outcomes also play a part in why we lack a good understanding of this area. For instance, we know that, compared to women with a normal BMI, women with a higher BMI have a higher chance of having a baby with a neural tube defect (NTD) such as spina bifida (Stothard *et al* 2009, Huang *et al* 2017, Vena *et al* 2022). But it is frustratingly difficult to find helpful data on the absolute risk of this. The chance of an NTD is low in the first place, so we need really big data sets to be able to see it, and we generally cannot know who is and isn't taking folic acid when we look at population-level data.

We do know that folic acid can prevent NTDs though, so all women are advised to take folic acid in pregnancy. It's possible that women with a higher BMI aren't getting enough folic acid, either because they need a higher dose and/or because they are dieting. But we don't know anything with certainty. Research into NTDs and BMI can tell us about the odds ratio, which describes the relative risk when we compare two groups. This is how we know that there is a difference in the relative risk experienced by women in different BMI categories. But I can't find enough of the right kind of data to be able tell you what the absolute risk is. Although, as Stothard *et al* (2009) explain, the absolute increase in risk with higher BMI is likely to be small.

Another issue which can complicate our understanding of whether and why women with a higher BMI are genuinely more likely to have a baby that has a congenital abnormality is that it can be hard to get good quality sonogram images in women with a high BMI (Pressman & Običan 2023). This means that anomalies may not be spotted in early pregnancy (Teale 2020), and parents may not discover their baby has an abnormality until later in pregnancy, or after birth. As a result, women with a lower BMI may be offered termination of pregnancy for a congenital abnormality at an earlier stage. There may well still be an increase in rates of congenital abnormality in larger women even if this were taken into account, but it is yet another illustration of how the data aren't nearly adequate or nuanced enough. We need better research.

Back to stillbirth and the bigger picture

I already looked at data on stillbirth at the beginning of this chapter, when I discussed relative and absolute risk. I want to return to this topic as I conclude this chapter. Hopefully, you now have a greater understanding that the adverse outcomes we are told are associated with higher BMI aren't always cut and dried. I discussed how it's important to look not just at relative risk, but also at absolute risk, as well as where the data come from. It's really important to analyse the studies rather than to assume that a guideline is necessarily correct or based on a fair evaluation of all of the relevant research. I've also discussed how guidelines may not take into account the underlying science, women's experiences, or the wider issues.

One of the forms of evidence most respected by health professionals is the reviews published in the *Cochrane Database of Systematic Reviews*. A Cochrane review is a systematic review of all the research on a particular topic, in which the reviewers use explicit, systematic methods that are designed to minimise the kinds of bias that can sometimes appear in research studies. Reviewers will focus on looking for the high-quality studies. The idea is that a Cochrane review will produce more reliable findings that can help to inform decision making. Knowing this can help us to see another aspect of the problem with guidelines. That is, sometimes, studies which aren't found to be of high enough quality to be included in a Cochrane review are still cited in guidelines and quoted to parents as evidence that being larger puts you 'at high risk'. It's worth being aware of that.

This isn't to say that I believe that randomised controlled trials, systematic reviews, and meta-analyses are the only useful kind of data. Nor do I think they are the best kind of study for answering every question that we might ask. I would say that all study results need to be considered and evaluated in a wider and broader context, which includes an understanding of the impact of our cultural beliefs, and how humans can affect research. But this kind of nuanced conversation isn't always what's happening in practice. That's another reason I want to finish this chapter with some reminders why we need to think very carefully about the data that are being shared on the topic of BMI and risk.

One issue is that some of the studies cited in the sections of the guidelines on stillbirth and BMI do not give us enough data to enable us to analyse the figures for ourselves. This is the case, for instance, in a study cited by the UK guideline on care for women with a higher BMI (Denison *et al* 2018) about stillbirth risk. The lead author on the cited study (Denison *et al* 2008) is also the lead author of the guideline itself. As was the case with the data on congenital abnormalities, the cited study gives us odds ratios for each category of BMI, which helps us to know about the relative risk, but it does not give us the absolute numbers. One reason that I would very much like to see the absolute numbers in this study is that there were also a lot of missing data (because BMI category at birth was not known), and there were far fewer women in the highest BMI categories than in the comparison group. This may be inevitable, as more people at that time were within the BMI range that the authors considered healthy, but missing data can make quite a difference to the results of a study.

It's also the case that, while some studies show higher rates of adverse outcomes for women with a higher BMI, others don't find this. For instance, Dalbye *et al*'s (2021) study of 7,189 first-time mums with a singleton fetus, cephalic (head down) presentation and spontaneous onset of labor at term found, *"No associations between maternal BMI and neonatal outcomes."* It's possible that these results have come about because it is a small study and we need larger numbers in order to see a difference in things that are thankfully rare. But I think it more likely illustrates how, if you have a higher BMI and your pregnancy progresses normally and labour starts spontaneously, then outcomes are equally as good as for those with a lower BMI. That idea is supported by other data that I will share later in this book.

Dalbye *et al*'s (2021) study also highlights the fact that we need better research to underpin the assertions that are made about neonatal outcomes, especially when we know that the way that women are treated may impact these outcomes. It's clear that many of the studies cited in the guidance and by professionals do not give us the full picture. This is probably also a good point to mention that studies which don't find a difference in things are less likely to be published. Or, if they are published, they are less likely to be cited in guidelines or in future studies.

When it comes to adverse outcomes for babies, the majority of studies do show that babies born to women in the very highest and lowest BMI categories are somewhat more likely to have a problem than babies born to women whose BMI is in the middle of the range. But there are a lot of problems with the research, which often doesn't take the wider picture into account. This makes it hard to give numbers for some of these outcomes. It's even harder to do this for women who are not of European descent, as most studies focus on this population.

As with other unwanted outcomes, the absolute chance of a women with a higher BMI experiencing a stillbirth or having a baby with a congenital problem is very low, and the vast majority of babies are healthy. Where studies show a correlation between higher BMI and adverse outcomes, we can't know whether this is a causative effect of higher BMI, due to issues in the research methods, to weight bias, to larger women and their babies receiving poorer care, to them being subject to additional tests and interventions which are having a negative knock-on effect, or to indirect factors that are associated with both higher BMI and these outcomes. We also know that there are some benefits to having a higher BMI.

But it's important to ask whether there is anything that we can do to prevent occasional but awful outcomes. In the next three chapters, I will discuss the tests and interventions that are offered to almost all plus size pregnant women in high-income countries to try to reduce or prevent adverse outcomes.

5. Pregnancy care and interventions

It is one thing to know that someone in one BMI category has a higher chance of experiencing certain outcomes than a person in another BMI category. But there are several other equally important questions that we might want to consider when deciding whether or not to take any action or accept recommendations that are offered as a consequence of this knowledge. The first one is to ask whether there is anything that can be done to reduce the chance of an adverse outcome, and also whether, as with pre-eclampsia or shoulder dystocia, there are things that can be done to treat it if the outcome occurs.

It's also critical to ask whether there is evidence that the things being offered are effective. We know that some of the interventions offered in maternity care are based more on tradition or fear of litigation than because they have been shown to be effective in well-designed clinical trials.

A further consideration is to weigh up the pros and cons of different courses of action to decide which is the best for you, as all interventions have potential for harm too. Finally, it can be useful to ask whether there are alternatives, and also to look at the wider context in which interventions are being offered. Sometimes, this can help us to understand why something is offered when a look at the evidence shows that it's not very effective, or there is perhaps no evidence to tell us whether it's effective or not. One reason people are offered interventions that aren't evidence-based is that, when faced with a problem, humans have a tendency to something called action bias. That is, we like to *do something* rather than just stand by and offer support or encouragement, even when the latter approach is known or thought to be more effective (Wickham 2022).

In this chapter, I look at the tests and interventions offered in pregnancy, with a view to helping answer some of these questions. There are a number of things that may be helpful to know if you decide that you do not want these things, or if you need help managing conversations to get your needs met. Rather than tell you the same things in each section, I have gathered them together in a tips section at the end of this chapter.

BMI and weighing as a screening test

Despite all of the evidence and recommendations that I detailed in chapter two showing that the current approach to weight, BMI, and health is inappropriate, unevidenced and harmful, obstetric guidelines remain focused on weighing women, calculating their BMI, and then offering advice and making recommendations based on this number.

NICE (2019a) removed the suggestion that women should be routinely weighed during antenatal appointments, because of a lack of evidence demonstrating any benefit coupled with concerns that this causes unnecessary anxiety. However, women in the UK still report being asked to step on the scales several times during pregnancy. The RCOG guideline states that, *"all pregnant women should have their weight and height measured using appropriate equipment, and their BMI calculated at the antenatal booking visit"* (Denison *et al* 2018). They also recommend that, *"consideration should be given to reweighing women during the third trimester to allow appropriate plans to be made for equipment and personnel required during labour and birth"* (Denison *et al* 2018). This latter point means that plus size women may be asked to step on the scales again in late pregnancy. It's up to you to decide whether this is right for you, though, and not the RCOG. I will return to this in the section on risk assessment consultations.

Weight measurement is also a routine feature of care in the USA (ACOG 2021) and it is recommended in Australia and New Zealand by RANZCOG (2022), who state that, *"All pregnant women should have a height, weight and BMI measured and recorded in their antenatal record at their first antenatal appointment, ideally before 10-12 weeks gestation. Weight gain in pregnancy should be monitored by re-checking weight at least once in each trimester."* The extent to which this guidance is actually followed does vary by practitioner and setting.

I've already mentioned how if you step on the scales during a medical or midwifery appointment your BMI will be calculated and used as a screening test to determine what care you will be offered. You have every right to decline. But it would be remiss of me not to mention situations in which you might need to be weighed. A key example is if you need or want certain medications, including a general anaesthetic. That's because dosages are calculated by taking someone's weight into account. If you decide to see an anaesthetist in pregnancy (as I discuss later in this chapter), you may find that they raise this. You may also be told you can't have certain antenatal screening tests if you don't step on the scales, which I'll also discuss below.

So you may need to weigh up the pros and cons of being weighed. It is possible to ask to be 'blind weighed', where you aren't told the figure. You can also ask for your weight not to be recorded in your notes, although it may not be possible to do this because electronic medical notes systems tend to pull data from other places. If, for instance, your booking weight wasn't filled out because you declined to be weighed but you then have a weight entered at 12 weeks because you want combined antenatal screening, you may find that this figure becomes your booking weight. It's also possible that someone looking at your notes later may see that your weight is missing and add it. They might even think they are being helpful, because they won't necessarily see that you explicitly asked for this not to happen. This is one of those unfortunate consequences of computer systems, bureaucracy and the way that systems of care are organised so that there is a tendency to treat everyone the same.

Antenatal screening tests

The antenatal screening tests which take weight or BMI into account include combined screening, which calculates the chance of your baby or placenta having certain problems or conditions, and non-invasive prenatal testing (NIPT). NIPT is a blood test that can give an estimate of how likely a baby is to have a chromosomal abnormality. It can also tell the sex of the baby and whether the baby is rhesus positive or negative.

In some areas, women have been told that they can't have these tests unless they consent to being weighed and having their BMI worked out, because the screening test calculations take weight or BMI into account. There is also a bureaucratic element to this. In England, for example, weight at the time of testing is one of the essential requirements on the data form used to order a NIPT test (NHS England 2021).

If you want to have antenatal screening tests but you are worried about the implications of being weighed then you may want to ask about this as soon as possible as these tests happen at set points in pregnancy, and the timing of when they are done can be important. You may wish to ask to speak to the screening team, who will have more in-depth and up-to-date knowledge about what is offered and possible in your area. Sometimes, for example, it is possible to have the ultrasound element of combined screening without having the blood test. However, in other areas having your weight recorded is non-negotiable if you want the screening as the computer programme contains fields that must be filled out for the calculation to occur.

It's also important to know that, if you have a higher BMI, there is more chance of a 'no call' result in a NIPT test (Juul *et al* 2020). This describes a situation where a result cannot be given, and it's usually because there weren't enough fetal cells in the blood sample that was taken from the woman. About 1 in 20 women with a BMI of 30-34.9 kg/m^2 have a no-call result, and about 1 in 10 women with a BMI of 35-39.9

kg/m^2 have a no-call result. In some studies, the chance of a no-call result was higher for women with a BMI of 40 kg/m^2 or more (Juul *et al* 2020). There is unfortunately nothing that can be done about this at the current time (Teale 2020), but you can at least be aware of this when you are deciding whether or not to have such tests. These types of tests cannot give certainty in any case, no matter what your BMI is.

Weight and diet-focused intervention

Several national recommendations include the suggestion that women's weight gain in pregnancy should be restricted (ACOG 2021, RANZCOG 2022). For example, the RANZCOG guideline includes a number of tables showing the amount of weight that women in certain BMI categories *"should"* gain, and states that, *"weight gain should be discussed and monitored regularly during antenatal care."* (RANZCOG 2022: 10). Their recommendation is that women with a higher BMI should gain less weight overall than women with a lower BMI.

This contrasts with the approach taken by the RCOG, who state that, *"there is a lack of consensus on optimal gestational weight gain. Until further evidence is available, a focus on a healthy diet may be more applicable than prescribed weight gain targets"* (Denison *et al* 2018).

It is true that some research shows that women who gain a very small or very large amount of weight in pregnancy may have a slightly higher chance of adverse outcomes (Goldstein *et al* 2017). But, as with the studies which look at outcomes in relation to a woman's BMI, it's not as simple as some people make it sound. The findings of individual studies vary, and there are multiple factors which may be influencing these results. It's also not that surprising that some women with lower weight gain during pregnancy have smaller babies and some women who gain more weight during pregnancy have larger babies. The baby's weight is part of their weight gain! It's also very unclear whether or to what extent weight gain itself is an issue, or whether both low/high weight gain and some adverse outcomes might be the result of something else, such as stress. This is particularly important when we consider women who have a relatively higher chance of adverse outcomes because of social and other factors, such as those living in poverty, and also for Black and Brown women, who experience racism and additional stress as a result of microaggressions.

But even if this were a clear and straightforward finding, as Denison *et al* (2018) point out, there is a lack of evidence to support the idea that it is beneficial to recommend limiting gestational weight gain or dieting in pregnancy. In fact, this is a rather problematic idea, as the entire point of pregnancy is to grow a baby, and babies have mass. If a baby weighs about 7-8lbs (about 3.5kg), and a placenta and amniotic fluid weigh another couple of pounds (just under 1kg) each, this adds up to 11-12lbs or 5-6kg by the end of pregnancy. Some babies are bigger than average, of course. Then there is the necessary increase in maternal blood volume, the size and musculature of the womb, changes in breast tissue, and the extra fluid and fat that the body stores as a vital, normal part of pregnancy.

It's also hard to be sure what constitutes an optimal weight gain in pregnancy. That's partly because we're all different shapes and sizes to begin with, but it's also because the whole idea of there being an 'optimal' weight gain is rooted more in cultural ideas about weight rather than health. I'm a bit loath to put a figure on the average weight gain in pregnancy here, because I don't want anyone to think I am saying that this is optimal, or something to aim for. But I want to emphasise that it is normal and healthy to gain a certain amount of weight in pregnancy for the reasons described above. So in that spirit I will state that, at term, the weight of the baby, placenta, amniotic fluid, and changes in the female body are likely to add up to 22-26lbs or 10-12.5kg. If you were taller or heavier in the first place, you may be at the upper end of that range.

But there's another issue, too. Even if limiting gestational weight gain (GWG) was a healthy, appropriate or evidence-based idea, a systematic review showed that, *"there is no optimal duration, frequency, intensity, delivery method, or diet for interventions aiming to prevent excessive GWG, making it impossible to definitively describe a tool box of 'best bets' that can be applied directly into practice settings"* (Walker *et al* 2018: 944).

A Cochrane review on this topic also found that although interventions including diet, exercise or both can reduce the chance of excessive GWG on average by 20% in the short-term, this made no difference to most outcomes (Muktabhant *et al* 2015). Again, as is common in birth-related research, most of the studies didn't look at medium or long-term outcomes for the women who were exposed to the interventions. I explained above how food restriction can mean that nutrient intake is decreased. This can have a number of negative consequences, as a pregnant woman's body will prioritise the baby's needs. This means that she can be left deficient in nutrients, which can increase the chance of a number of physical and mental health problems. There is a worrying lack of discussion of such issues in research studies and the documents that describe the care of pregnant and postnatal women.

However, even when evidence shows that recommending dieting or limiting GWG isn't beneficial or effective, some recommend these things anyway, both in practice and in the medical/midwifery literature. This is another demonstration of action bias. In one example, a senior Australian obstetrician acknowledges the lack of research and yet still calls for action:

"While it has proven difficult to limit weight gain in many RCTs, meta-analysis supports the need to at least attempt to adhere to weight gain advice with subsequent potential reduction in a variety of pregnancy complications." (Teale 2020)

The authors of such statements often seem to be saying that, while we don't have good evidence that limiting weight gain is beneficial, and even though we know that diets don't work, it would be nice if they did, so let's recommend them anyway. Another example of the gulf between the evidence and what happens in reality is that, even in the UK where the recommendation is to avoid focussing on weight gain targets, these limits are still being imposed on women.

"When I worked in a large obstetric unit [in the UK] we had a BMI clinic as part of the pathway, where all women with a BMI over 30 are sent. It still happens. It's really humiliating for them. They get extra scans and a glucose tolerance test. The stated aim is that they maintain their weight and not put any more on. I've never found out if there's any real evidence for this. You can see they are triggered at being put down and patronised." (Amanda, midwife)

The issue is that, given the essential increase in mass that is an intrinsic part of pregnancy, being told to not put on weight during pregnancy is tantamount to telling you to lose weight, or at least to diet. The only way of growing a healthy baby without putting on weight is if you lose the same amount of weight from your own frame. This is even more problematic as an idea given what I previously wrote about how your body needs to adapt to pregnancy as well. It begs the question of whether one reason that plus size women have a slightly higher chance of experiencing adverse outcomes is because they are being told to restrict what they eat and to follow unevidenced guidelines rather than to listen to their own bodies and follow their own instincts around how to nourish themselves.

Some of the weight-loss interventions offered during pregnancy are quite worrying. Blaylock *et al* (2022) surveyed pregnant women and, somewhat shockingly, found that:

"Several survey respondents also reported their data being shared with third parties, such as Slimming World, which further undermined trust between them and their midwife:

'Because of my weight (high BMI) I was offered an additional service about losing weight which I did not want, I declined and it still was pushed on me and she turned up to my appointment without my consent' (survey respondent)." (Blaylock *et al* 2022)

Midwives and women from around the world have shared their concerns with me about this aspect of antenatal care for plus size women.

"In Australia, women are sent to a group. They call it 'fatty club'. It does nothing except perhaps help them bond with others in

a shared experience of group fat shaming. I'm not sure that's the stated aim." (Rachel Reed, midwife)

Amanda, who I quoted above, also explained that, *"Many of the women who were coming in* [to the high BMI clinic] *knew more about diets than me, and they were following the diets but it seems like the diets themselves don't work. I felt that the clinics were damaging to their self-esteem. I disliked doing that pathway because I knew I was going to be putting people through pain."*

I want to add an important note about the assessment of women's experiences of weight loss and dietetic services, antenatal groups and special clinics just for women who have a higher BMI. These continue to run because researchers find that they are *"well liked"* (Tyson *et al* 2022). I don't doubt that some women enjoy these and find them useful, although the same researchers also note that others don't feel this way. My own inbox and those of size friendly colleagues is full of emails from women who feel shamed and humiliated in such settings, and dread going to them almost as much as they dread the judgement they can receive if they don't go.

It's not hard to imagine why such variation in viewpoints exists. We're all different, and some women would like to lose weight and feel supported in such a setting, while this may not be the case for others. Women report feeling that they had to pretend to like the groups in order to be seen to be trying to lose weight. Others, as Rachel noted above, find support in a mutual experience of something unpleasant, which begs concerning questions. It's possible that the women who dislike this approach are among those who don't return their surveys to researchers (and we know that the response rate in such studies is often poor). They may also not tell the truth:

"So yeah, I said it was good on the form because I was worried they might get social services on me, but it literally was awful. Humiliating. I used to feel sick before going. It was probably the worst bit of being pregnant." (Sally)

We need far more research into women's experiences (Hoch *et al* 2023), which vary considerably. Although I don't have space to look at it separately in this book, we know that body image is related to gestational weight gain and weight stigma (Hill *et al* 2023), and this is likely to be an issue for some women when weight loss clinics and groups are advised. That's an important note to end this section on, because the issues discussed in this section are a key area of distress and even trauma for some women.

Although I have explained in this section that there isn't evidence to support weight and diet focused interventions in pregnancy, the key take-home message is the same as it has been throughout this book. It's your body, and your baby, and the important thing is that you weigh up your individual situation and the options that you are offered, and then decide what is right for you. Please also see the tips section at the end of this chapter.

Folic acid and vitamin D

I mentioned in chapter four that women with a higher BMI have a higher chance of having a baby with a neural tube defect (NTD). As with many adverse outcomes, the absolute chance of this is still very low. Dwyer *et al* (2022) summarise:

"Neural tube defects, which include spina bifida, anencephaly and encephalocele, are ... estimated to affect 18.6 per 10 000 [which is 1 in 538] *live births worldwide; 50% of cases result in elective terminations or stillbirths."*

One way of further reducing the chance of having a baby with an NTD is to take folic acid, and we have good evidence that this is effective (De-Regil *et al* 2015). As with so many interventions, we don't have such good data on possible downsides, and it's always your decision, of course. In most countries it is recommended that all women take folic acid for three months before becoming pregnant, if possible, and then for the first 12 weeks of pregnancy. The recommended dose is 400µg per day.

In many areas, women with a BMI of 30 kg/m^2 or higher are advised to take a higher dose of folic acid over the same time period. The recommended higher dose is 5mg per day.

Just to put this into context, 5mg is the equivalent of 5000μg, so larger women (and some other women perceived to be at higher risk of having a baby with an NTD) are being told to take 12.5 times the standard dose. The reasoning for the higher dose being offered to women with a higher BMI is the higher chance of having a baby with a neural tube defect. It is true that people who weigh more do need higher doses of some medicines for them to be effective. However, this is another example of where a focus on BMI rather than weight may be unhelpful, because a shorter woman with a BMI of 32 can easily weigh less than a taller woman with a BMI of 28. Therefore, you may wish to take this into account when deciding whether or not to take a higher dose of folic acid.

Furthermore, the advice to take a higher dose of folic acid is not an evidence-based recommendation, and that's because there is no evidence on this topic. As Dwyer *et al* (2022) explain, *"We lack evidence to suggest that high doses* [of folic acid] *have additional benefit in preventing neural tube defects in women with other risk factors."* They also discuss the, *"lack of evidence on benefits or harms of high dose folic acid."* Some women feel that they would rather take the higher dose in order to ensure that they are doing everything possible to reduce the chance of NTDs. Only you can decide what's right for you.

Several countries' guidelines also recommend vitamin D supplementation for those with a higher BMI. For instance, the RCOG guidelines state that:

"Obese women are at high risk of vitamin D deficiency. However, although vitamin D supplementation may ensure that women are vitamin D replete, the evidence on whether routine vitamin D should be given to improve maternal and offspring outcomes remains uncertain." (Denison *et al* 2018)

As Vestergaard *et al* (2023) discuss, it isn't uncommon for pregnant women to be lacking in vitamin D and there is some evidence that vitamin D may help reduce the chance of some adverse outcomes, including pre-eclampsia and gestational diabetes, but more evidence is needed. Additional studies are underway (Vestergaard *et al* 2023).

Although women often ask about dietary sources of folic acid and whether being in the sun can give adequate vitamin D, we don't have good evidence on these questions either. The lack of good evidence when it comes to folic acid and vitamins means that it will likely come down to you weighing up your individual situation, family context and personal beliefs in order to determine the decisions that are right for you.

Aspirin for the prevention of pre-eclampsia

In chapter four, we saw that higher BMI is one of a number of factors known to be correlated with having a higher chance of developing pre-eclampsia. Many genetic and other factors play a part in this as well (Townsend *et al* 2019). Pre-eclampsia is, for instance, less commonly seen in women of Asian descent (Burton *et al* 2019) and more common in women who have ancestry from sub-Saharan Africa (Nakimuli *et al* 2014). I also explained that we have effective ways of diagnosing and managing pre-eclampsia. But pre-eclampsia can sometimes lead to serious complications, especially if it is not diagnosed and monitored, and some women who have pre-eclampsia will be advised to have their baby delivered early. Much focus is now being placed on whether and how we can predict or prevent it (RCOG 2022).

Townsend *et al* (2019) highlighted that higher BMI and weight are the factors most strongly predictive of pre-eclampsia, but it's important to understand what that does and doesn't mean. It doesn't mean that pre-eclampsia is inevitable if you're overweight, and it doesn't mean that BMI is the only or most important factor. But BMI is very easy to measure. So if you have a treatment that you think can help prevent pre-eclampsia and are trying to reduce the number of women who get pre-eclampsia on a population basis, then targeting women with a higher BMI or other risk factors is a relatively simple means of trying to achieve your goal.

In the past few years doctors have begun to prescribe some women daily aspirin in the hope of reducing their chance of developing pre-eclampsia. If you have a BMI of 35kg/m^2 or more then the increased chance of developing pre-eclampsia may mean that you are offered low dose aspirin during pregnancy (usually a daily dose of 150mg from 12 to 36 weeks). Sometimes, women with a BMI under 35kg/m^2 are offered low dose aspirin, especially if they have another risk factor, such as being older, being pregnant with their first baby, or having a family history of pre-eclampsia.

At the time of writing, doctors and midwives are not in agreement about the use of aspirin to prevent pre-eclampsia. Low dose aspirin isn't licenced for use in this way in some countries, including the UK, and it's clear that we need more and better research. However, its use is supported by the National Institute for Health and Care Excellence (NICE 2019b). Early trials showed that low dose aspirin was not beneficial when given to all women in pregnancy (Rotchell *et al* 1998) but studies which focus on women who are at higher risk of pre-eclampsia have shown that low dose aspirin may have benefits. More research is under way, and other medications are also being investigated (Ma'ayeh & Costantine 2020). Currently, the best evidence summary is a Cochrane review which helpfully explains the numbers.

"Administering low-dose aspirin to pregnant women led to small-to-moderate benefits, including reductions in pre-eclampsia (16 fewer per 1000 women treated), preterm birth (16 fewer per 1000 treated), the baby being born small-for-gestational age (seven fewer per 1000 treated) and fetal or neonatal death (five fewer per 1000 treated). Overall, administering antiplatelet agents to 1000 women led to 20 fewer pregnancies with serious adverse outcomes. The quality of evidence for all these outcomes was high.

"Aspirin probably slightly increased the risk of postpartum haemorrhage of more than 500ml, however, the quality of evidence for this outcome was downgraded to moderate, due to concerns of clinical heterogeneity in measurements of blood loss. Antiplatelet agents [which include aspirin] *probably marginally increase placental abruption, but the quality of the evidence was downgraded to moderate due to low event numbers and thus wide 95% CI*

[confidence interval]. *Overall, antiplatelet agents improved outcomes, and at these doses appear to be safe. Identifying women who are most likely to respond to low-dose aspirin would improve targeting of treatment. As almost all the women in this review were recruited to the trials after 12 weeks' gestation, it is unclear whether starting treatment before 12 weeks would have additional benefits without any increase in adverse effects. While there was some indication that higher doses of aspirin would be more effective, further studies would be warranted to examine this."* (Duley *et al* 2019)

Offering aspirin to pregnant women deemed to be 'at higher risk' of pre-eclampsia is a good example of a prophylactic intervention that is offered because it works on a population basis where the absolute number of women who benefit is very small. Bear in mind that, while women with a higher BMI are often told they are 'at high risk' here, the figures I shared in chapter four show that around 87% of women with a BMI of 35 kg/m^2 or higher won't develop pre-eclampsia. Most of those who do develop it will not experience serious problems, but pre-eclampsia can lead to very serious complications in a small number of cases, and is occasionally fatal. This again underlines why it's important to weigh up the pros and cons as they relate to your situation, as different decisions will be right for different people.

In another example of how we need to look more widely, Mollard *et al* (2023) found that taking exercise, getting more sleep (which included napping) and greater vegetable consumption prior to pregnancy are all associated with a lower chance of pre-eclampsia in first-time mothers. The researchers didn't break down the results according to BMI, but none of these things can do harm and they are simple factors which may help reduce the chance of pre-eclampsia.

In fact, midwives have been discussing the importance of good nutrition and self-care in preventing and treating early signs of pre-eclampsia for as long as I can remember. Many of the things that they recommend have now been shown to be effective in studies. A useful summary of the research linking nutritional intake and a reduction of pre-eclampsia risk was shared by Perry *et al* (2022). They found evidence of benefit for eating at least 400g of fruit and vegetables per day, getting plenty of fibre, eating vegetable oil, and limiting foods high in fat, sugar and salt. Beneficial nutrients include calcium, a daily multivitamin/multimineral supplement, and ensuring that you have adequate vitamin D. If people have a low selenium intake, they may benefit from eating more fish and seafood or from taking a supplement. Some benefit has also been seen from milk-based probiotics (Perry *et al* 2022).

Restricting food groups can cause problems here as well. We know, for instance, that people's blood pressure can be raised if they don't get enough potassium. This is especially the case if they eat a lot of food containing sodium, which is found in salt. Yet some of the most readily available sources of potassium, which include bananas, sweet potatoes and potatoes, are the very foods that some of the weight loss programmes and GDM diets tell people to avoid. Could the fact that women with a higher BMI have a higher chance of developing pre-eclampsia be partly to do with the greater likelihood that they have been dieting? We have no evidence either way, but it's an interesting question. This is another example of how the notion that there are 'good' and 'bad' foods can be really unhelpful. There is, again, a bigger picture here, and other avenues that may be worth exploring.

Gestational diabetes screening and treatment

There has been a huge amount of discussion and debate about screening and treatment for gestational diabetes (GDM), but there is very little that we can be sure about. GDM is of concern because it is associated with an increased chance of some complications, including pre-eclampsia, macrosomia (which I discuss below), neonatal hypoglycaemia (low blood sugar in babies), and an increased chance of some long-term health conditions (USPSTF 2021).

However, several aspects of this debate are controversial.

Definitions, screening and suggested treatment vary widely, the increased chance of complications is small, and there is very little evidence that either screening or treatment are beneficial (Farrar *et al* 2017, Tieu *et al* 2017, Martis *et al* 2018). There are also data showing that early screening does not improve outcomes (Champion *et al* 2022), and there is no consensus on whether or how we should be offering screening or treatment (Hegarty 2020, US Preventive Services Task Force *et al* 2021).

In some countries, including the USA (ACOG 2021) and Australia (Australasian Diabetes in Pregnancy Society 2014), all pregnant women are offered screening for GDM, but women with a higher BMI may be offered this at an earlier point in pregnancy. In other countries, including the UK, testing is offered only to women deemed to have a greater chance of developing GDM. This includes women with a BMI of 30 kg/m^2 or higher, those over 40, women of south Asian, Black, African-Caribbean or Middle Eastern origin, and women with a history of GDM or family history of diabetes (Denison *et al* 2018).

The screening test given to women with a higher BMI is called an oral glucose tolerance test (OGTT) and is designed to see how your body copes with sugar. It involves having your blood tested for sugar levels before and after having a special sugary drink. You will usually be asked to fast for a few hours beforehand and then attend a clinic where your 'fasting blood' will be taken. You'll be given the drink, asked to wait two hours and then have your blood taken again.

Many women report disliking the OGTT.

"Women discussed … the difficulties of undertaking the OGTT. Lived experiences were shared, particularly when reporting their dissatisfaction of the OGTT (having time off paid employment, childcare arrangements, and physical effects from the test). Results from the survey demonstrated that 56% of women felt nauseous during the OGTT." (Shipton *et al* 2022)

One in five women who have a BMI of 35 kg/m^2 or more will have a positive result on an OGTT test (O'Dwyer *et al*

2012). They may be offered interventions as a result, and yet a look at the evidence highlights many uncertainties in this area. Cochrane reviewers looking at whether it is effective to screen for GDM according to risk factors (including BMI) concluded that we do not have enough evidence to know whether screening based on risk is effective (Tieu *et al* 2017). This is also the finding of reviewers who looked at screening for GDM in general and concluded that, *"we are uncertain about which strategies to diagnose GDM are better, as we have assessed the quality of evidence as very low. Large randomised trials are needed to establish the best way for identifying women with GDM."* (Farrar *et al* 2017)

The state of our knowledge about treatment for GDM is summarised by the authors of another Cochrane review:

"Currently there is insufficient high-quality evidence about the effects on health outcomes of relevance for women with GDM and their babies for many of the comparisons in this overview comparing treatment interventions for women with GDM. Lifestyle changes (including as a minimum healthy eating, physical activity and self-monitoring of blood sugar levels) was the only intervention that showed possible health improvements for women and their babies. Lifestyle interventions may result in fewer babies being large. Conversely, in terms of harms, lifestyle interventions may also increase the number of inductions. Taking insulin was also associated with an increase in hypertensive disorders, when compared to oral therapy. There was very limited information on long-term health and health services costs. Further high-quality research is needed." (Martis *et al* 2018).

As Martis *et al* (2018) note, one of the biggest risks of having GDM screening is that you may find yourself under pressure to accept interventions, including earlier induction of labour. I will return to induction in more depth later, but the key thing to know at this point is that there is no evidence suggesting that induction is beneficial for women who have GDM. A Cochrane review found only one small trial which showed no benefits to induction. More of the babies born after induced labour had jaundice, though (Biesty *et al* 2018). An Australian study found that women who had GDM but no other specific medical conditions were more likely to have a caesarean if their labour was induced at 38, 39 or 40 weeks compared to women who had expectant management (Seimon *et al* 2022). The World Health Organization advise against induction for gestational diabetes alone (WHO 2018).

I also want to mention Metformin, which is a medication sometimes offered to women with a higher BMI or a diagnosis of GDM. In the UK, women who have been diagnosed with GDM will be advised to change their diet and be more active. If dietary change doesn't work to maintain their blood sugar within the target range, they will be offered Metformin. In some areas of the world, Metformin is offered instead of dietary changes. Cochrane reviewers who researched this concluded that, *"there is insufficient evidence to support the use of metformin for women with obesity in pregnancy for improving maternal and infant outcomes. Metformin was, however, associated with increased risk of adverse effects, particularly diarrhoea"* (Dodd *et al* 2018). Diarrhoea can potentially impact the absorption of nutrients and vitamins.

There is a great deal that we do not know about GDM, and this is a reason to tread carefully when making decisions. A recent study highlighted that the incidence of GDM varies by season (Stalheim *et al* 2023), which is an intriguing finding. The rate of GDM is lower in the summer months and, while this research cannot tell us why this is the case, this finding begs the question of whether GDM is linked with vitamin D, women being able to get outside more, eating more fresh vegetables/salad, or something else that occurs differently in the summer months. Another reminder that we need to look outside of the current paradigm and think more widely.

Given the state of our knowledge, and the above findings about the interventions that are currently offered in response to a diagnosis of GDM, some women question whether they want to be screened for this at all. Others feel it is worthwhile because if they know early on that they have an issue with insulin they can at least manage that. There's a school of thought which suggests that, because none of us actually need refined sugar from a physiological perspective, eating refined sugar is something that any woman can opt out of if she wishes to avoid GDM screening while limiting her chance of developing GDM-related problems. I want to be clear that, as with the conversation about nutrition and pre-eclampsia, this option isn't about dieting or weight loss. As Julie Frohlich, a Consultant Midwife summarises, *"it's about not putting too much strain on your pancreas, and respecting the complex dance that goes on in your body around resistance to insulin."*

If you would like to know more about this topic in general, both Rachel Reed (2018) and I (Wickham 2023) have freely available online resources.

Screening for macrosomia (big babies)

There is no evidence that screening for macrosomia or offering induction of labour in the hope of preventing it (which I discuss in chapter six) is effective. We cannot know the birth weight of a baby for certain until it is born and placed on a set of scales, but we do know that screening for big babies and offering induction can cause harm (Wickham 2021a).

One significant problem is that, while professionals have tried to estimate a baby's weight during pregnancy for many years, it turns out that this is very difficult, and we are often wrong. I have written a lot about this in one of my previous books, so I'm going to quote myself here.

"Measuring babies in a woman's womb with our hands or with a tape measure is accurate only half the time (Chauhan et al 2005) ...ultrasound isn't very accurate at predicting a baby's size either. Most studies and reviews show that there is a margin of error of 15% either way (Rossi et al 2013, Boulvain et al 2016, Milner & Arezina 2018)." (Wickham 2021a: 118)

"So for a baby estimated to weigh 4kg ... a 15% margin either side means the range of the estimate is from 3400g (7lbs 5oz) to 4600g (10lbs 4oz). That's quite a range. And it's still only an estimate, not a guarantee. A few babies will weigh more or less than a weight that falls within the 15% margin. Curiously, professionals

seem more likely to overestimate than underestimate. The researchers in the 'Listening to Mothers' survey … found that one in three women were told their baby was 'too big' based on ultrasound, and yet the actual average birth weight of the babies who were suspected of being big was 7lb 13oz or 3590g (Cheng et al 2015)." (Wickham 2021a: 119)

Part of the problem is that our current means of screening for macrosomia are incredibly crude and don't take factors such as maternal size or genetics into account. Most of the studies are based on limited local populations, but it's also unhelpful to pool it together. For example, Bhattacharya *et al* (2007) looked at outcomes of women who gave birth in Aberdeen between 1976 and 2005. The researchers don't give data on ethnicity or heredity, but it's highly likely that the vast majority of the women were white. Similar studies have been done in many other countries around the world, based on populations living locally. This poses a challenge to anyone trying to share data in a way that will be useful to everyone because, as we saw in chapter two, socioeconomic factors (Gaudet *et al* 2014, Zeng *et al* 2023) and ancestry (Harvey *et al* 2021) can make a big difference when it comes to measures like BMI and birth weight. Large differences in nutrition, maternity care, and socioeconomic and educational status exist around the world, and there is a concerning lack of data from Africa, Asia and South America (Gaudet *et al* 2014).

Women of Asian descent are particularly disadvantaged because they and their babies are often being measured against growth charts that use figures based on populations of predominantly white women or on mixed populations. Problems can be missed or over diagnosed.

These problems aren't easily solved and they wouldn't necessarily lead to better methods anyway. We need to accept that there are things that we cannot accurately predict, and that our attempts to do so can lead to more harm than good.

Ultrasound scans

All women nowadays are offered ultrasound scans in pregnancy, usually including a dating scan, combined screening, and an anomaly scan. It's common for women with a higher BMI to be offered extra scans during pregnancy, called serial growth scans, and sometimes an additional scan in late pregnancy. In fact, many other women are now being offered these as well, but I'm going to focus on how these are offered to plus size women.

Ultrasound scanning is a really interesting technology because many women look forward to scans and find them reassuring, but they can also be the source of a great deal of anxiety. Lots of people aren't aware that scans are not a perfect technology and that they have a high margin of error, as I discussed in the section on macrosomia. The inaccuracy is acknowledged in some guidelines (Denison *et al* 2018) and yet scan measurements are still treated as being reliable and have become a routine aspect of care. They are also often the starting point for recommendations for further monitoring (including more scans) and interventions such as induction.

One thing I want to mention about scans in general is that, if you have a higher BMI, they can be more difficult to do. You may be asked to move or hold your tummy, so that the sonographer (the person doing the scan) can get the probe in the right place, and the operator may need to press a bit harder than usual. This means that it may take a bit longer or on occasion you may be offered a repeat scan.

It is also possible that the sonographer will ask to do a transvaginal scan. This question is sometimes asked during the scan itself, so you may want to consider whether or not you want this ahead of time. The word 'transvaginal' means through the vagina, so this is an internal examination. A transducer (or probe) is inserted into the vagina so that the internal organs and baby can be visualised. Women and midwives tell me that these are frequently offered to larger women. We don't have much data on safety or effectiveness, and risks include discomfort, pain, and infection (Hamm *et al* 2020). It's always up to you whether you want any sort of scan or not. You can decline a transvaginal scan and request to just have an abdominal scan.

You may want to think about what clothes you wear, so you can give the sonographer access to your body without feeling cold or exposed. You can take someone for support. If you are told that this isn't allowed, you have the right to leave or ask for a different appointment to which you can bring a support person. Some women report feeling bruised after a scan, but having a scan should not hurt. Remember that you can ask the sonographer to stop at any time.

Let's begin with anomaly scans, which are routinely offered to all women at around 20 weeks of pregnancy. Anomaly scans are designed to look for any problems that your baby might have, so that you can be directed to specialist care (for instance fetal medicine or intrauterine surgery), make neonatal care plans, or be offered termination of pregnancy if severe problems are detected. I mentioned in chapter four that congenital abnormalities are less likely to be picked up in women with a higher BMI, and this is partly because scans are less accurate in larger people. Teale (2020) adds that *"it is worth warning of the frequent need to repeat the investigation which can be time consuming and anxiety provoking."*

Many women with a high BMI are offered serial growth scans. The timing of these can vary a bit between areas, but a common pattern in the UK is to offer them at 28 and 36 weeks. The 36 week scan is sometimes instead called a late pregnancy scan or third trimester scan. In certain countries, women are offered scans more frequently, and sometimes at every visit.

The reasons often given for the use of serial growth scans or late scans are that (a) there is an increased chance of macrosomia and (b) that measuring the size of the uterus with a tape measure (symphysis pubis height measurement) isn't as accurate when someone's tummy is bigger. I've already discussed macrosomia in chapter four, along with the fact that measuring the size of unborn babies isn't very accurate in anyone, no matter their size or shape, so you might question why ultrasounds are used so often. I question that too, but again the answer is probably that we don't have anything better, and action bias means we perceive it is better to do something than nothing.

A group of researchers (Neel *et al* 2021) looked specifically at the use of a growth scan between 34 and 36 weeks of pregnancy in women who had a BMI of 35 kg/m^2 or higher. Neel *et al* (2021) noted the estimated birth weight recorded in the scan and then compared this with the actual weight of babies at birth. The results were very interesting, but I need to explain a couple of terms before I describe what Neel *et al* (2021) found.

I mentioned in chapter two that, when researchers look at something we call 'sensitivity', we are talking about measuring how effective a screening test is for finding all the people who have a disease or problem. Ideally, we want tests that find a high number of 'true positives', or the people who have a problem. This is especially important as tests may have risks and downsides themselves, including creating anxiety. It's also helpful if a test is specific, or has high specificity, because that means we are not identifying lots of people as potentially having a problem when they actually don't.

Unfortunately, Neel *et al*'s (2021) study again highlighted the problems that occur when we try to use scans to predict which babies will be large or small. But the issues are different for large and small babies, so let me explain one at a time.

As has been the case in other studies, Neel *et al* (2021) found that the sensitivity of ultrasound scans for predicting which babies are small for gestational age (SGA) was poor. Scans only identified 8.1% of the babies who were actually small for gestational age. The good news is that the specificity for predicting SGA babies in this study was 100%, so they didn't incorrectly identify any babies as being SGA when they weren't. (It's not always 100%. This is just one study.)

When it comes to predicting which babies will be large for gestational age (LGA) on late scans, we have a different problem. Neel *et al*'s (2021) data show that scans correctly predicted 61% of the LGA babies, which is a better rate of true positives than for SGA babies. However, the specificity (or positive predictive value) for LGA babies was 54.8%, which means that only 54.8% of the babies which scans predicted to be LGA were actually large at birth. Nearly half of the parents who were told their baby was predicted to be LGA didn't go on to have an LGA baby.

Overall, only 40% of the actual birthweights of the babies in this study were within ten per cent of their estimated birth weight according to the scan. Neel *et al* (2021: 116) concluded that routine third trimester ultrasounds were of *"limited utility in helping identify aberrant fetal growth."* I would say that this is putting it mildly, especially when you consider another key finding of this study was that *"46% of ultrasounds overestimated fetal weight by >10% when compared with the actual birthweight percentile."* (Neel *et al* 2021: 120).

What this means is that nearly half of the women with a higher BMI who have a scan in the third trimester are told that their baby is more than ten per cent heavier than it actually is when born. This is an important finding because ultrasound scan results play a key part in leading to a recommendation for induction of labour. I have heard from many women who are frustrated that an incorrect ultrasound prediction was used to persuade them to abandon their birth plans and accept interventions that they didn't want. This is why decisions about whether or not to have scans are actually far more important than many people realise.

When it comes to tests like ultrasound, it's important to be able to tease out why you're being offered something. Some offers of testing or intervention are genuinely individualised, but many things are recommended to everyone. Some tests are offered to all women who fall into a certain category, and that's not really any different to them being recommended to everyone, because it's still not about you as an individual. It's about the fact that you have a BMI over 35 kg/m^2, or your blood pressure is a certain number, or you have reached a particular point in your pregnancy. That's not individualised.

It's always up to you to decide whether or not you want a test or intervention, ideally after receiving good, evidence-based information from someone who is focused on helping you make the decisions that are right for you and your family. It can be really helpful to work out whether something is an individualised recommendation, something that's offered to everyone, or something that's offered to everyone who is in a particular category that you happen to fall into. And it's always worth considering the downsides, and the fact that agreeing to a scan or other screening tests may lead to a false diagnosis or an outcome you don't want.

Heparin injections

I discussed in chapter four that higher BMI is one of the risk factors that can increase someone's chance of having a venous thromboembolism, or VTE. So, in many countries, VTE risk assessment is carried out at one or more points during pregnancy, birth and the postnatal period. Depending on where you live, you may be offered injections of low molecular weight heparin (LMWH) during pregnancy in the hope of reducing the chance of a VTE. Although low molecular weight heparin is only one type of heparin, I'm going to use the word heparin in this book when I'm talking about low molecular weight heparin for ease of reading.

The list of risk factors for VTE is actually quite long, and it varies a lot between countries. Some risk factors are seen as more important than others, and the criteria for being deemed 'at high risk' change at different stages of pregnancy and the postnatal period. In most countries, you won't be offered heparin during pregnancy unless you have had a blood clot in the past or you have an inherited condition known as thrombophilia, which you will likely already know about. In the UK, however, some women with a higher BMI are offered heparin injections in pregnancy. The scoring system used to assess for VTE risk means that women are sometimes surprised that they are being offered heparin, so it is worth getting informed about what this is, and the issues that relate to it ahead of time.

In the UK, pregnant women with a BMI of 30 kg/m^2 or more who also have other risk factors will be offered heparin in pregnancy. These other risk factors include having had a blood clot in the past, having recently had surgery, being a smoker, being older, having a higher BMI, having had three or more babies before, and having *"gross varicose veins"* (RCOG 2015). Some women are offered heparin from early pregnancy and some from 28 weeks, depending on the number and type of risk factors.

Once your baby is born, a slightly different set of risk factors is used, which I will discuss in chapter seven. The higher chance of experiencing a VTE in the postnatal period means that, once the baby is born, it only takes one risk factor in addition to having a BMI over 30 kg/m^2 to mean that you are offered heparin for prevention of VTE if you're in the UK. Similar scoring systems are used in other countries, and they're relatively easy to look up online.

Low molecular weight heparin is an anticoagulant. This means that it thins your blood and thus makes blood clots less likely. It is known by a number of different names, including Dalteparin (Fragmin®), Enoxaparin (Clexane®, Inhixa®), and Tinzaparin (Innohep®). Heparin can be broken down by stomach acids, so it has to be given by injection, usually once or twice a day. If you decide to have heparin, you will be taught to give yourself the injection. Heparin doesn't cross the placenta (Flessa *et al* 1965, Harenberg *et al* 1993), so it is considered the safest anticoagulant to give in pregnancy. Although warfarin can be given in tablet form, it can cross the placenta and cause harm to a baby.

Side effects of heparin include bruising at the injection site, an allergic reaction, and an increased chance of bleeding. This can include minor bleeding, such as nose bleeds and bleeding more if you cut yourself by accident, but more serious kinds of bleeding can also occur, especially during and after birth.

This means that women who decide to have heparin in pregnancy will be strongly advised to birth in hospital and have medical management for the birth of their placenta. They have a greater chance of bleeding from their uterus, a tear or caesarean section wound, or of having a haematoma, which occurs where blood pools in one area (Lu *et al* 2021). This can be a problem if someone who has heparin in pregnancy has an epidural in labour, as an epidural haematoma is serious. For this reason, anaesthetists will not site an epidural if insufficient time has lapsed since a heparin injection. Midwives and doctors will try to plan the timing of heparin injections with the risk of bleeding in mind. So women will be advised to stop giving themselves the injections at the first sign of labour, or before they come to hospital for an induction, but birth isn't always predictable. There are also some rare side effects of low molecular weight heparin, including abnormal potassium levels and a type of abnormal immune reaction called heparin induced thrombocytopenia (HIT).

The use of heparin is controversial, both in pregnancy and the postnatal period. When one looks at the guidelines which discuss the risk assessment strategies and the preventative treatment for VTE, they are again based on expert opinion rather than evidence. Yes, we know that some groups of people have a higher chance of having a VTE than others, but the idea that anyone with a particular number of risk factors should be offered heparin isn't evidence-based.

The lack of evidence to support offering heparin for risk factors is acknowledged by a number of obstetric associations. The American College of Obstetricians and Gynecologists (ACOG), for instance, explains that no widely accepted risk scoring system has been tested or validated and we have no evidence to tell us whether having more than one risk factor has any impact on someone's chance of developing VTE (ACOG 2018). They have concluded that there is poor evidence for offering heparin in pregnancy unless women are genuinely at high risk because they have a history of VTE or a thrombophilia (ACOG 2018).

As most of the conversation on heparin is based around offering heparin in the postnatal period and I don't want to repeat things too much, please see the section on VTE and heparin in chapter seven for a deeper discussion of the issues and the evidence. As I explain in more depth there, we don't have good studies on whether heparin is effective, even if someone does have risk factors. Heparin came to be used in the UK after VTE was shown to be a leading cause of maternal death. And while the number of deaths is very small, their impact on families and caregivers is life altering, so it's understandable that guideline making organisations and health care professionals want to try to do whatever they can to prevent VTE. But there's still no evidence for most of what is currently being recommended, and we can't be sure it does more good than harm.

As a reminder, the data I shared in chapter four from a study by Butwick *et al* (2019) showed that, during pregnancy, VTE was experienced by 1 in 2632 women with BMI of 25-29.9 kg/m^2, by 1 in 2380 women with BMI of 30-34.9 kg/m^2, by 1 in 2128 women with BMI of 35-39.9 kg/m^2, and by 1 in 943 women with BMI 40 kg/m^2 or more.

As I will also discuss in chapter seven, there may be other things that you can do to lower your chance of VTE. These include not smoking, getting up and moving often, being well hydrated, and not crossing your legs when sitting. Using compression stockings (flight socks) may help prevent DVTs in the legs, although they don't prevent all types of VTE.

A key risk factor for VTE in the postnatal period is having had a caesarean. So you can also reduce the chance of VTE after birth by doing everything you can to prevent a caesarean. This might include planning where you will give birth, who will care for you and be with you in labour, and learning how you can maximise your chance of staying mobile, avoiding unnecessary interventions and having a straightforward labour and birth.

Risk assessment consultations

Some plus size women find that they are being assessed in late pregnancy, often without prior notice, in something called a 'moving and handling risk assessment'. This is another practice that is encoded in guidance but for which there is no evidence beyond the opinion of those who wrote the recommendation.

"Women with a booking BMI 40 kg/m² for whom moving and handling is likely to prove unusually difficult should have a moving and handling risk assessment carried out in the third trimester of pregnancy to determine any requirements for labour and birth. Clear communication of manual handling requirements should occur between the labour and theatre suites when women are in early labour. Some women with a booking BMI less than 40 kg/m² ...may also benefit from assessment of moving and handling requirements in the third trimester. This should be decided on an individual basis." (Denison *et al* 2018)

In Blaylock *et al*'s (2022) survey of women's experiences of pregnancy-related public health advice and risk messages in the UK, *"Approximately 26% (n= 1841) of survey respondents reported feeling judged because of their weight and described dehumanisation and depersonalisation within the maternity care system. This is exemplified by one woman who was present for conversations about how staff would move her should she become incapacitated in labour:*

'I accept that there is also the risk of the idea of my body as an object which is large. Therefore [it] *poses a risk to staff who are handling my body. That is a very depersonalising way to think about oneself. I'm aware that is something that has to be considered, but I feel quite strongly that risk needs to be considered in private and not in front of me.'"*

It's clear that such conversations are not always handled well. We need to question whether they are warranted in the way that they are happening in systems of health care. It's also the case that there are some things that need to be different when women have a very high BMI. There is, for example, a need to ensure that staff are trained in safe manual handling, though this should happen across the board. Some equipment has weight limits, and it may be important to ensure the availability of appropriate lifts or hoists, longer surgical instruments, wider operating tables, and correctly sized surgical stockings and pneumatic compression devices (both of which help to prevent DVT). We know that care needs to be taken when larger people have surgery. Caesareans can take longer and different positioning may be needed (Neel & Teale 2019). But it could be argued that these things should be available at all times, given that a greater number of people have a higher BMI these days, and that hospitals should be prepared to look after anyone at short notice.

Plus size women may be offered appointments with an obstetrician and anaesthetist to discuss this and other issues, so let's look at these next.

Obstetric consultations

In countries where you see a midwife for most or all of your antenatal care, plus size women are sometimes given one or more appointments with an obstetrician as well. Many women are happy with this and do not question it. I am including this conversation in this book for those women who were not happy about this experience, or who wished they had known that they could decline such appointments.

The nature, purpose and pattern of appointments depends very much on where you live. In some areas, all women are offered an appointment with an obstetrician, and this is a routine occurrence during pregnancy. In others, referral to an obstetrician is based on having a risk factor, which can include a higher BMI. So if you are not sure why you are being offered an obstetric consultation, then ask. Once you find out the purpose of the appointment, and whether it is a routine offer or based on an actual concern about your or your baby's health, you can decide what to do. It's also important to ask whether you are actually seeing a consultant, or one of their team who will have varying degrees of experience.

One of the reasons that some larger women have found obstetric appointments difficult is that their decisions were questioned. Some report feeling coerced into changing their mind about having a home birth, going to the midwifery led unit, or declining induction of labour. Others felt they were 'steamrollered' into unwanted intervention, although this can also happen in appointments with midwives and other health care professionals. As with many of these decisions, the important thing is to consider your own situation, for instance whether you are healthy and having a straightforward pregnancy, or whether you are experiencing problems or have concerns about your health.

Anaesthetic consultations

In many areas, women with a BMI of 40 kg/m^2 or higher are also given an appointment with an anaesthetist during pregnancy. This is so the anaesthetist can assess you, in case you need or want an epidural, spinal or general anaesthetic during labour. It is true that, if someone has a high BMI, having a general anaesthetic carries a greater chance of problems (Cook *et al* 2011). This is why it can be better to have regional anaesthesia, which means an epidural or spinal anaesthetic, if you have a caesarean. However, it can also be trickier to put one of the needles used for a spinal or epidural anaesthetic into someone's back if they are larger. If someone has a very high BMI or has poor health in other ways then they may need specialised equipment to be used if they need surgery. One reason for the appointment is to discuss these issues so that you are informed, and so that any specific needs can be assessed and recorded.

During the appointment, you'll be asked about your health, for instance whether you experience sleep apnoea. The anaesthetist may ask to examine your neck to assess your airway and your back, to see whether they might need a longer needle if you wanted or needed an epidural or spinal anaesthetic. They may also ask to look at your hands and arms, to assess how they would insert a cannula if you needed intravenous fluids.

If you have previously declined weighing, they may ask you to be weighed in case you need a general anaesthetic. However, it's still your decision. The reality is that, if a pregnant woman is admitted to a hospital in an emergency having had no antenatal care and needs an immediate caesarean, or if someone with a high BMI needs surgery after a car accident, the anaesthetist will manage the situation without knowing their exact weight. In fact, anaesthetists are actually very good at estimating what dosage someone needs. On the other hand, it can be safer and more relaxed for everybody if the conversation happens ahead of time and they have accurate information about you.

You may find that the anaesthetist offers advice and recommendations, and suggests a pain relief plan for labour and birth. In fact, guidelines recommend that *"an anaesthetic management plan for labour and birth should be discussed and documented. Multidisciplinary discussion and planning should occur where significant potential difficulties are identified"* (Denison *et al* 2018). Remember that guidelines are for health professionals to follow, though. It is up to you whether or not you agree to any suggestions.

There are pros and cons to this type of risk assessment. The midwives I spoke to when I was writing this book differed in their views on how worthwhile an anaesthetic assessment is for plus size women. Some feel this is a conversation worth having, in case you do need an anaesthetic in a hurry. If you have questions or concerns, then a knowledgeable and kind anaesthetist can help you weigh up the pros and cons of different options in one appointment.

On the other hand, some women found the conversations they had with anaesthetists to be unhelpful and full of weight bias that they would rather have avoided. Some midwives report that women often see a less experienced member of the team and mentioned that the chances of seeing the same doctor in labour are slim. They questioned the value of having a physical assessment when the doctor on duty at the time would need to perform their own assessment rather than rely on notes made by a colleague. As with obstetric consultations, some women who plan to give birth on a midwifery led unit or at home have found it undermining to have someone try to talk them out of it, particularly when scare tactics are used.

Some anaesthetists recommend a 'just in case' epidural. This is so that, if an emergency caesarean is needed, an effective regional anaesthetic is already in place and (a) they won't have to take on the additional risks of giving someone a general anaesthetic or (b) spend the extra time that it can sometimes take when putting an epidural into someone who is larger than average. And it does sometimes take a bit more time; that's not in question. Epidurals aren't always effective, and it's also true that some women do need to have a caesarean in a hurry. But most of these 'emergency caesareans' aren't emergencies in the same way that a fire is an emergency, and there is usually time to put a spinal or epidural in. It's also the case that epidural anaesthesia will limit your ability to move around in labour, which itself may increase your chance of needing a caesarean (Goer 2022).

Another issue raised by a number of midwives is that it may be important to distinguish between well and unwell women, and for you to consider your own weight, mobility and general health when deciding if you want to attend risk assessment appointments. Decisions are often best made in the context of someone's individual situation. A key issue for some women is whether they can see an anaesthetist who will be supportive, kind and respectful of them and their decisions, or whether they will encounter weight stigma or a risk-focused approach that isn't aligned with their needs. You can ask whether you have a choice in who you see. Your midwife may be able to give you more information about this. There are some very kind and respectful anaesthetists out there, and this is exactly the kind of situation where different decisions will be right for different women.

Risk, restrictions and resolutions

Many plus size women are told in pregnancy that they will not be 'allowed' to birth in a midwifery led unit or to use a birth pool in labour. I'm going to go into more depth on what we know about the issues relating to these options in chapter six, but I've mentioned them here because, if you want to birth in a midwifery led unit, use a birth pool or do anything else that your caregiver seems to think might not be possible or advisable because of your BMI, you would be well advised to start addressing this and looking for solutions as early in pregnancy as possible. There are a number of reasons for this. One is that you might not have so much energy later, and it can sometimes take several conversations to get what you want. Another is that, if you are told that you can't have these things, you may want to look at other options.

These options include hiring a pool for early labour or planning a home birth; no-one can stop you from getting into a pool or bath in your own home. In fact, there's no guarantee that you will be able to use a pool that's in any kind of unit anyway, no matter what your BMI or risk status. It may not be available, or someone else might be using it. You can always decline care, as long as you are conscious and have capacity, but you don't always have the legal right to insist on certain things. *What's Right For Me?* (Wickham 2022) looks at this in more depth if you would like to explore it further. But let's also look at some ways of negotiating what you want or need during pregnancy.

Negotiating what you want or need

It's often possible to negotiate what you want or need within the local maternity care system, and I've included this section to offer some suggestions on how to do that.

It's important to understand that both you and your health care providers have rights *and* responsibilities. Health care providers are legally obliged to give you certain information and, if they are employees within a system or bureaucracy, they may not have as much power as you might think they do. It's really frustrating to be told you can't have or do something, but if you stay calm and ask questions which will help you understand where the decision making power lies and why there is a barrier, you will often get further as you'll know where to target your efforts. Sometimes care providers really want to help you, but you might also need to help them, for instance by taking responsibility for a decision rather than asking them to endorse or offer an option that is outside of what their employer or the local guidance says they can offer.

Clearly explain what your needs and requests are. It can help if you take evidence (for instance this book) and clearly demonstrate that you are aware of the concerns (even if you don't agree with them) and have thought through the pros and cons of different options.

Make notes of conversations so that you have a record of who said what and when. Ask for letters that summarise your discussions at appointments with health care providers.

If you are told that you can't access the type of care you want, reiterate why you are asking, and ask the health professional what other options you have. Explain why you're asking (even if you feel you're repeating yourself), and why what they are offering doesn't meet your needs.

Explain to the care provider that you are willing to take responsibility and sign a waiver if this would help.

Be wary of health professionals who tell you to 'wait and see'. This may sometimes mean that they're hoping to find some way of making the issue go away, perhaps by raising the question of other risks later, or waiting until you're in early labour and have less energy or ability to be assertive.

Anticipate potential derailment. Women who plan an out-of-hospital birth may be told that a late scan has highlighted a problem, for instance that their baby seems big. This may or may not be a genuine concern, but it is worth bearing in mind that it happens, and being prepared for it if it does.

If you are not getting anywhere, you may want to consider

whether the birthplace or care provider is right for you, or whether there are other options that you might look into.

If you are otherwise happy with your chosen place of birth or you don't feel you have any other options, ask to speak to a consultant midwife, a manager or, if you're in the UK, the Head of Midwifery.

Writing an email or letter can be effective, especially if you copy key people in. Look online to see who is in charge of the hospital or service, and who regulates health or maternity services in your area.

Seek independent support locally; this might be from a patient advisory service, a local support or home birth group, or a birth worker such as a childbirth educator or doula. There are often patient support services, advocacy groups or people who support those trying to get the care they need. It's worth doing research to see if there are any in your area.

The tips on managing conversations at the end of this chapter may help as well.

What isn't being offered?

In this chapter, I discussed the care and interventions that are offered during pregnancy in the hope of preventing unwanted outcomes in women with a higher BMI. Given some of what I've written in previous chapters, one might think that care would also be taken to offer things that would optimise physiology, reduce weight stigma, and help solve the problems faced by plus size women. Yet this isn't happening. At every turn, the focus is on unproven interventions that often lead to other interventions, which may be more likely to cause problems, rather than on lower tech alternatives. Often, long-term risks of interventions haven't been researched.

I discussed preterm birth earlier in chapter four, noting that the data on this vary, so we can't be certain whether women with a higher BMI are at more or less risk of this. There is another deep irony when it comes to preterm birth, however. The one thing that is known to reduce the chance of having a preterm baby is midwifery-led care (Sandall *et al* 2016). Yet many plus size women are being immediately directed into obstetric-led care simply because of their BMI, and regardless of how healthy they are by any other measure. This means that they are missing out on the many advantages of midwife-led care, which also includes having less chance of losing their baby (Sandall *et al* 2016).

I mentioned the effect of setting, carer and care in chapter four, but I'm going to raise it again, because it could be that at least part of the increase in unwanted outcomes in plus size women is the result of the care that they are getting, and the fact that they are missing out on individualised, midwife-led care during pregnancy.

I am also concerned that, while we know that having a higher BMI during pregnancy is associated with a greater likelihood of experiencing depression (Marchi *et al* 2015, Ruhstaller *et al* 2017, Dawe *et al* 2020), little is being done to address this. This is particularly worrying given everything I wrote about weight discrimination in chapter two, and the fact that maternity services are singling out larger women in ways that women find to be stigmatising, depersonalised and judgemental rather than supportive (Furber & McGowan 2011, Blaylock *et al* 2022). Black and Brown women and their babies are at even greater risk, as I have already noted.

We know that plus size pregnant women may experience feelings of self-doubt about their ability to give birth (Knight-Agarwal *et al* 2016). Risk management increases stress, fear and anxiety, and can have a negative impact on outcomes and experience (Wickham 2004, Haines *et al* 2012, DeJoy and Bittner 2015, Coxon *et al* 2016 Rodrigues *et al* 2016). Anxiety disorders in pregnancy are associated with preterm birth, hypertension, pre-eclampsia, caesarean section, and a number of other unwanted outcomes (Coehlo *et al* 2011, Ding *et al* 2014, Buckley 2015, Nagl *et al* 2015, Dunkel Schetter *et al* 2016, Ravid *et al* 2018). But we are not addressing this. This again also begs the question of how much of the problem is the way we treat those with a higher BMI rather than their BMI itself, yet those with a higher BMI are being channelled into the very interventions that can increase the chance of a problem, or of experiencing more intervention.

It can sometimes seem as if the maternity services are so focused on trying to manage the risks associated with higher BMI that women often aren't given the kinds of information, advice and support that would actually be useful to them, and that can help manage pregnancy on a day-to-day basis.

One key piece of advice that you may not be told by risk-focused maternity care providers is to be aware that it might take longer to feel your baby kick, and that advice on baby's movement and other aspects of pregnancy experience is often geared around the experience of women with a BMI in the average range. It's worth spending time relaxing with your baby and your body, finding ways to be kind to your body, and learning about your own pregnancy and what feels good for you and your baby.

Some women who have a higher BMI benefit from and enjoy aqua exercise groups, swimming, or just spending time in water. This can help with movement and mobility, and it can reduce stress. If you don't enjoy swimming in mixed groups, there are sometimes women only or plus size friendly sessions. This also applies to yoga and stretching groups if you think you might enjoy those. The key is to find ways of moving your body that work and feel comfortable for you.

There are a number of forums for larger women where you can get tips and share experiences, and some plus size women find these to be supportive. But please be aware that some of these groups are very medically or diet culture focused, while some are run by people seeking to profit from selling information which may or may not be accurate, so it's worth doing your research before deciding whether to join.

It is also worth looking outside of what is offered within the maternity services to see if there are people, groups, or services that could help you in pregnancy. I realise that not everybody can afford to hire support, but some services can be accessed for free or at low cost, so it's worth doing some research to see what's available in your area. There are now also lots of people you can follow online but, again, do some research. Find out about their background (are they qualified?); their approach (are they kind, judgemental, diet focused?); and their goals (support, ego boosting, community, pure profit from selling 'tools' that might undermine your confidence, making a living while helping people?) before you decide who you will allow to influence your journey.

I am going to end this section with a few tips that I have picked up over the years for managing the conversations that I deeply wish you didn't need to have.

A few tips for managing conversations

As I wrote this book and talked to women, friends and colleagues, I gathered a few tips for avoiding or managing conversations about weight management, weighing or other tests or interventions should you decide you don't want them.

I offer them here for you to adopt, adapt, ignore, or use as a basis to help you think more deeply about what you might need or want from your health care providers.

You may wish to prevent the conversation coming up unexpectedly by telling the person at the beginning of the encounter that you do not want to be weighed, discuss your weight or have a particular intervention. A useful sentence can be, *"I'm aware that you may be obliged to raise the question of BMI, but I don't want to discuss it, thanks."* Some people prefer to wait and see if it comes up (and more on that below), but others would rather address it at the outset.

If you'd rather wait and see what happens, you can simply answer any question about whether you would like a conversation about your weight with *a 'no, thanks'*, or just *'no'*, which is of course a complete sentence. You can respond the same way to any direct question offering you a weight-related conversation or intervention.

Sometimes the opening to a conversation will be phrased

in different ways, so be prepared for that. Have a few possible responses ready. A professional may say: *"We need to discuss your weight/BMI"*, *"How do you feel about your weight?"*, *"What are you doing to lose weight?"*, or *"Tell me about your diet"*. Sadly, some are less polite. Some will make reference to their own weight and size, as if that makes it more okay to talk about yours. Some will be apologetic, and some will acknowledge that it is your decision to talk about it or not.

Remember that you can almost always change your mind at a later date, or re-initiate a conversation that you previously decided that you didn't want to have. So if you aren't sure, it may be better to say you need time to think.

Other useful phrases include, *"I don't want to discuss that"*, *"I'm not interested"*, and *"That's not something I want to go into"*.

In every case, remember that you can always take a moment before you respond.

If the health professional or birth worker repeats the same question, let them finish and then repeat your answer. It can be more effective to simply keep saying *"No, I don't want that"*, than to be drawn into a discussion.

Remember that you are not obliged to explain why you don't want something.

If you need more time to think, or think a question was phrased rudely, ask for the question to be repeated. It will give you a moment to think, and it may also cause the person to reconsider their words. As the wonderful midwife Mary Cronk used to suggest, you can say something like, *"I don't think I can have heard that correctly. Could you please repeat that?"*

If you are being asked something that you aren't sure about or consider inappropriate, you can also ask the person to repeat it so that you can record it on your phone. You can always say that you want to discuss it with your partner later.

If you are worried that you will feel nervous and forget key phrases, write down what you want to say beforehand and keep it in your hand or on a post-it on your phone.

By the time you get to the end of this book, I hope you'll feel more confident about what you do and don't want and with what the evidence actually says. If you're worried you'll forget something, many people take my books to their appointments, sometimes bookmarked with sticky notes.

There are a number of people who have also written good books and websites or who you can follow on social media. Reading more will help you become more confident in your understanding, and that will help you to advocate for yourself in such situations.

Finally, there are information sheets and handouts that you can print out and give to health professionals to let them know that you don't want to discuss weight or weight loss strategies. You might want to keep some of these handy. You can find these and other resources at www.lindobacon.com.

6. Care during labour and birth

One of the key things that defines western medicine is that it takes a compartmentalised, linear, and focused approach to defining and treating diseases. This is in contrast to looking at the person as a whole, and considering the wider issues. In theory, in western medicine, we determine (diagnose) what the problem is, and then we recommend a particular drug, intervention, or treatment. So if someone has high blood pressure, we might offer medication to lower blood pressure. If you have a headache, you get a painkiller, and if you've broken a bone then, depending on the severity, you might be offered orthopaedic surgery. But in all of these cases, there's a clear link between the problem and the offered solution, and these clear links are what makes randomised controlled trials a good way of measuring the effectiveness of western medical treatments. When we can clearly define who has the problem (for instance anyone with a systolic blood pressure of more than 140mmHg), we can randomise them to having a blood pressure pill or a placebo, measure the outcome and easily see whether or not the pill is effective at lowering their blood pressure. The same is true when care or intervention is offered to you by a health professional. We think you have problem X, so the solution we are offering is Y. Here's our rationale, here's the evidence, do you have any questions, and what would you like to do?

This theoretical ideal is unfortunately not always what happens in the care of plus size women. There are some interventions that I write about in this book, and blood thinning drugs are a good example, which are offered in the hope of preventing a clearly defined and potentially serious problem; in this case, VTE. You may or may not want to have them, when you weigh up the evidence and your situation, but the rationale for them is clear. But in quite a few of the situations where extra tests, interventions, and restrictions are offered to women with a higher BMI, things are less clear, and are sometimes confusing. Some women find they are given several different reasons to justify the same intervention, and induction of labour and care during labour in general is an excellent example of where this happens. The fact that someone can cite several reasons for having something does not necessarily mean that the intervention is more justifiable, urgent, or beneficial. In most cases, there is absolutely no research into whether having multiple risk factors affects your chances of experiencing an unwanted outcome.

When it comes to intervention around labour and birth, you may sometimes notice that the reason given for doing something is unclear, or that it changes or seems illogical. You may decline something that was recommended for one reason, but then find you are told there is now another reason that you need the same intervention. It's not uncommon, for instance, for women to find they are given several reasons to justify induction, which I will discuss in the next section. Some women decline an offer of induction which is based on their age, for example, only to be told that it is recommended because of their BMI. If they decline again, they may be told that there are concerns about the size of their baby, their blood pressure, or something else. This doesn't happen to everyone, of course, and I hope it doesn't happen to you. There are some good reasons for induction, but offers of induction aren't always evidence-based (Wickham 2021a). A similar thing can happen with electronic fetal monitoring (EFM), augmentation (speeding up labour with an oxytocin drip), and advising instrumental birth or caesarean for slow progress.

In this chapter, I'm going to look at some decisions and interventions relevant to labour and birth. Some of these are offered for reasons other than higher BMI, of course, or for multiple reasons, which is why I began by explaining this issue. But the principles are always the same. You have every right to ask for evidence and take time to consider what's right for you. There is another tips section at the end of this chapter with more information on this.

Induction of labour

As I explained above, women with a higher BMI may be offered induction of labour for multiple reasons. The offer may be made simply on the basis of their BMI. It may be made because they are also a bit older, because they might have gestational diabetes, because there is concern that their baby may be bigger than average, or because they have pre-eclampsia. Sometimes, a few of these are cited at the same time, and this list isn't even exhaustive.

I'm going to quote myself a lot in this section. That's because I've written a PhD thesis and two books on induction, so I have a lot of material to draw on. As an overall summary, I can tell you that, while there is sometimes evidence of a slightly increased chance of stillbirth or adverse outcomes in some of the situations where induction is offered, the absolute chance of stillbirth remains small. More importantly, there is often no evidence that induction makes a difference. But induction is associated with a higher chance of other adverse outcomes for mums and babies, including caesareans, other interventions, and long-term negative consequences.

I want to mention the relationship between induction and caesarean. You may have heard, or you might be told, that induction decreases your chance of caesarean. This is occasionally true, but only if you are a participant in a very medically-focused clinical trial which includes a narrow population of women and criteria specific to that trial (Wickham 2021a). If you give birth in the real world, induction increases the chance of caesarean (Davey & King 2016, Zhao *et al* 2017, Levine *et al* 2021). It also leads to longer labour, more interventions, and means you're likely to be in hospital for longer (Wickham 2021a, Ellis *et al* 2019).

You are even more likely to experience negative consequences from induction if you have a higher BMI. Ellis *et al* (2019) found that caesareans were more common for women with a higher BMI who had an induction compared with women who had a BMI in the 'normal' range and whose labours were induced. The women in the studies they analysed who had a higher BMI also had longer labours, were given more drugs during their induction, and the induction was more likely to fail (Ellis *et al* 2019).

The fact that induction is more likely to lead to caesarean than when labour is allowed to begin spontaneously is of particular concern, because plus size women have a higher chance of problems when recovering from caesareans (Denison *et al* 2018). For this reason, it seems logical to try to reduce the chance of caesarean as much as possible, especially in women giving birth for the first time. A key way of doing that is to save induction for when it is truly warranted, and to not offer it when there isn't genuine evidence of benefit (O'Dwyer *et al* 2013).

Induction and pregnancy length

It's important to know that a woman with a higher BMI is more likely to have a longer pregnancy than someone with a lower BMI (Denison *et al* 2018, Slack *et al* 2019). This can mean that more women with a higher BMI are advised to have induction for post-dates pregnancy relative to those with a lower BMI. But both pregnancy length and BMI have a genetic element, so longer pregnancy may simply be a familial tendency and 'normal for them'. It's difficult to be sure about this, partly because women with a higher BMI are also more likely than women with a lower BMI to be given an inaccurate due date if they have a scan to date their pregnancy (Källén *et al* 2013, Kullinger *et al* 2016). This is particularly ironic and frustrating as we know that larger women have more scans.

It's also worth bearing in mind that, when women with a higher BMI are told that their baby is large for its gestational date, it may well be the ultrasound scan gestational date that is wrong. Not to mention that babies vary in size. The existence of lots of uncertainties mean that, if you are offered induction based on your baby's gestational age, or your baby's size as predicted by ultrasound, you may want to remember that there is a wide margin of error with both. If, for instance, you are certain of your conception date, you may not want to accept an ultrasound 'guesstimated due date' that is different.

One reason that it's particularly important to ensure that your baby is not born too soon, either by induction or elective caesarean, is that *"babies of high BMI women* [born by elective caesarean before 39 weeks] *were particularly prone to the need for assisted ventilation (help breathing) and treatment in the Neonatal Intensive Care Unit"* (Vincent *et al* 2018). Any baby born too early is at risk of needing such care, which is why induction and elective caesarean need careful thought, but babies born to women with a higher BMI may be at particular risk. It's possible that a baby's size and gestational age are more likely to be estimated wrongly in plus size women. Although evidence clearly shows that larger women may have longer menstrual cycles and thus longer pregnancies (Wickham 2018, 2021a), this unfortunately seems not to be well known by medical practitioners, and it isn't accounted for in obstetric guidelines.

One final thing is that plus size women are sometimes told that they need more monitoring if their pregnancy progresses 'post-dates'. We have no evidence about whether this is useful or not, as it has not been studied. It may well lead to more intervention, and women report that monitoring appointments are frequently used to try to persuade them to accept induction.

Induction for maternal BMI

Women with a higher BMI have long been told that they need their labour induced because of their size (Cedergren *et al* 2004), despite a lack of evidence showing that this is beneficial. When it comes to induction for maternal BMI:

"There are no randomised controlled trials that have looked at outcomes relating to larger women and induction of labour. So we don't have any robust evidence to tell us whether or not induction

is beneficial for larger women or their babies. Some researchers are calling for randomised controlled trials to look at induction in larger women (Coates et al 2020, D'Souza et al 2021). Given the problems in the trials that have looked at induction for post-term pregnancy, suspected macrosomia and older maternal age, however, it is difficult to be sure that any trial looking at induction for larger women would tell us anything except that this group of women are also more likely to be told they need a caesarean, whether or not this is the case by any objective measure.

"We do have some data from retrospective studies, which look back at women's medical records to see what happened in different groups of women, but the results are very mixed and not very reliable. In some hospitals, larger women who had induction were less likely to be told they needed a caesarean than women who received expectant management (Lee et al 2016, Glazer et al 2020). But in others the chance of caesarean was the same for larger women no matter whether labour was spontaneous or induced (Kawakita et al 2017). Several studies found that induction increases the chance of caesarean in larger women (Wolfe et al 2014, Ruhstaller 2015, Little et al 2019, Carlhäll et al 2020, Hamm et al 2021). Most of the studies show no difference in outcomes or do not look at this. The results of those that do show a difference vary. Pickens et al (2018) found fewer adverse outcomes in babies born to larger women who had induction. By contrast, Wolfe et al (2014) found that the babies born to larger women (with a BMI of 30 or more) whose labours were induced were more likely to be admitted to neonatal intensive care. It's very difficult to draw any conclusions when the results vary so much between studies. We should also bear in mind that all larger women are at risk of being told they need intervention in mainstream maternity care. In Dalbye et al's (2021) study, larger women in spontaneous labour were more likely to be told that they needed a caesarean or that their labour needed to be augmented, or speeded up with drugs. In addition … most of these studies are American and are based on a very medicalised approach to birth. The samples aren't representative of larger women in general and, again, outcomes are affected by professional decisions." (Wickham 2021a)

At least one study on induction at 39 weeks of pregnancy in plus size women is underway (Krogh *et al* 2021), but there is every chance that it will be beset by the same biases as many of the other trials that have been carried out to evaluate the use of induction of labour (Wickham 2021a).

Induction for gestational diabetes

Some women are told that they need to be induced because they have GDM. However, there is no evidence showing that induction is beneficial for women with gestational diabetes, and this applies to women of any BMI.

There has actually only been one small trial on induction for GDM. It included 425 women and their babies, compared induction of labour with waiting for spontaneous labour, and it showed no difference in outcomes between women whose labour was induced and women who waited for labour to start spontaneously. As the Cochrane review summarises:

"The findings of this trial highlighted no clear difference between the babies of women in either group in relation to the number of large babies, baby's shoulder getting stuck during birth or babies with breathing problems, low blood sugar and admission to a neonatal intensive care unit. No baby in the trial experienced birth trauma. In the group of women whose labour was induced, there were more incidences of jaundice in the babies." (Biesty *et al* 2018).

In the UK, NICE (2020) recommend that earlier induction (or elective caesarean) should generally not be offered to women solely because of GDM unless either the mother or baby is experiencing complications. This should be a genuine medical problem and not just a risk factor, and a number of other authors express concerns about the recommendation for induction for GDM given the lack of evidence of benefit (Jabak & Hameed 2020) and the fact that this results in more caesareans (Seimon *et al* 2022).

Induction for suspected macrosomia

I've already discussed the fact that we cannot accurately predict which babies will experience shoulder dystocia, a situation which occurs in about 1 in 150 term births (RCOG 2012). Our inability to accurately predict shoulder dystocia is acknowledged in guidelines (RCOG 2012). However, this hasn't stopped many women from being advised to have their labour induced because of a fear of it happening. This advice is not based on good evidence (Wickham 2021a), but the frequency of this recommendation may be because, while serious consequences of shoulder dystocia are very rare, they are one of the most common reasons that parents take legal action against doctors and hospitals (RCOG 2012).

I previously looked at the evidence for induction for a suspected big baby, and concluded:

"there are serious flaws in the idea of offering induction for a suspected big baby. It isn't supported by the evidence. We can't accurately predict the weight of a baby. Even if we could, weight isn't directly correlated with the chance of shoulder dystocia, and most babies who experience shoulder dystocia are fine. Most babies who are larger than average will be born easily, especially if their mothers are able to move about as they want to and have the kind of care which helps optimise the physiology of labour.

"There's just no evidence that screening for macrosomia, telling women that their baby is thought to be larger than average (while omitting to mention that there is a margin of error in the estimation) and offering induction when a baby is suspected to be larger than average is helping. But there is plenty of evidence that these practices are causing anxiety, stress, trauma, morbidity and harm." (Wickham 2021a)

A worrying new trend exists where obstetricians are recommending induction in situations where a baby's abdominal circumference is estimated to be above the 90th or 95th centile. There is no evidence to support this practice, which is not cited in any national guideline that I can find. It is of particular concern given the 15% margin of error for ultrasound at term, which I have already discussed. This intervention isn't only being offered to women with a higher BMI but plus size women are often offered serial growth scans, so they may be offered induction for this reason.

Another concerning issue is an Australian study which *"showed that, for a woman having her first baby, the chance of having a caesarean after induction varied according to the reason for induction (de Vries et al 2019). In that study, the women most likely to end up with a caesarean were those whose labours were being induced for a suspected large baby"* (Wickham 2021a). It may be that in some cases these babies were genuinely unable to be born through their mother's pelvis, but we don't have good evidence that this is the case, and there are many other factors that need to be considered. The uncertainties in this area give us even more reason to look not just at reducing unnecessary and unevidenced inductions, which can lead to poorer outcomes, but at how we can help women to optimise their physiology during labour and birth.

BMI and place of birth

Although plus size women are often told that they need to give birth in a hospital, I doubt you will be surprised to read that there are discrepancies in the guidelines and a lack of evidence to support this idea as well. In the UK, as just one example, one section of the RCOG guidance acknowledges that having a BMI of 30-35 kg/m^2 isn't in itself an indication for hospital birth, but then later states that the 'additional care' that a hospital can offer should be discussed (Denison *et al* 2018). The NICE (2022) guidance recommends hospital care for women with a BMI of 35 kg/m^2 or more, but fails to provide robust evidence to support this, and ignores the evidence that I discussed in chapter four which shows that some larger women have equivalent and sometimes better outcomes when they birth at home or in birth centres, and with care providers who believe in them (Hollowell *et al* 2014, Rowe *et al* 2018).

In research, it's often difficult to separate out the impact of place of birth and care provider approach on outcomes. That's because home births are almost always attended by midwives rather than doctors, and midwifery-led units are by definition staffed by midwives. But that doesn't matter for our purposes. The key issue is that there is generally less focus on risk management and routine intervention when women labour and birth at home or in homelike settings, which may also help explain why women who choose them often have better experiences and outcomes. More on this in the section on labour progress.

As I discussed in chapter three, two key studies on this topic have been carried out in the UK. I make no apology for looking at them again here, because they are so important in helping us understand the deeper issues that can help women to make the labour and birth decisions that are right for them.

As a reminder, Hollowell *et al* (2014) looked at women with a higher BMI who gave birth in different settings. They found that women who were healthy, had given birth before, and had a higher BMI were at lower risk of having a problem in labour than had been previously thought. Their results didn't support the idea that healthy multiparous women with a higher BMI should give birth in hospital. This is why Hollowell *et al* (2014) suggest reviewing the BMI criteria for planned birth in non-obstetric settings, which would make birth centre and home birth more accessible for those women.

But why do they not make the same recommendation for women having their first baby? Well, mainly because we know that the chance of having a problem is a bit higher when it's your first baby, across all settings, and so guidelines are worded more cautiously when it comes to place of birth for first-time mums, regardless of BMI. But if you are considering home birth, then you're probably already aware of the issues, and I can tell you that I have not found evidence that higher BMI alone will particularly increase your chance of a problem. I certainly know of and have attended many healthy women who had a higher BMI and who successfully, safely, and joyfully had home births. Including Sofia from chapter one.

The second important UK study is the UKMidSS Severe Obesity Study (Rowe *et al* 2018). Data were collected from all of the 122 alongside midwifery units (AMUs) in the UK at that time. The outcomes of larger women were compared with the outcomes of women with a BMI under 35 kg/m^2. The women who had had a baby before and whose BMI was between 35 kg/m^2 and 40 kg/m^2 were no more likely to need intervention or to have an adverse outcome than other women who had given birth before and who had a lower BMI. In other words, they aren't at increased risk, and 96% of these women had a straightforward vaginal birth (Rowe *et al* 2018).

So BMI again makes no difference in outcomes for women who have had a baby before. When it comes to women having their first baby, there was a slightly higher chance of women with a BMI of 35-40 kg/m^2 experiencing birth interventions or adverse outcomes compared to women with a BMI of less than 35 kg/m^2, but most of these outcomes were things that can be easily treated and the researchers couldn't be sure whether the difference was significant. A key fact from this research is that 67.9% of the women with a BMI of 35-40 kg/m^2 having their first baby in a midwifery-led unit had a straightforward vaginal birth. Considering the high caesarean rates that exist today, this is an impressive percentage.

Given the results of these two studies and everything else I've said so far about the risks associated with intervention, we might well ask why UK women with a higher BMI aren't being offered care in midwifery-led units, or other midwifery-led environments. It is inequitable that, as I illustrated by detailing the different experiences of Sofia and Ana in the introduction to this book, healthy women with a lower BMI are being offered the chance to birth in midwifery-led units, while women who are equally healthy and simply have a higher BMI are being actively discouraged from doing this, or denied this option altogether. When we realise that the women who opt for hospital birth have a higher chance of complications and intervention, which can mean they face increased risks in later pregnancies, it is hard to understand how policymakers and clinicians can think that such recommendations are justified.

The UK isn't the only country in which out-of-hospital settings have been shown to be advantageous to plus size women. In a study of larger women who gave birth in birth centres in the USA, the majority again experienced an uncomplicated pregnancy and a straightforward vaginal birth. They experienced no more complications or adverse newborn outcomes than women with a lower BMI (Jevitt *et al* 2021). The researchers concluded that healthy women who have a higher BMI *"can receive safe and effective midwifery care at freestanding birth centers while anticipating a low risk for cesarean birth"* (Jevitt *et al* 2021: 14).

I want to add another finding for anyone who has a higher BMI and GDM and is advised to have a hospital birth for this reason. Researchers looked at whether there was evidence to support a recommendation for hospital birth for those with GDM. It turns out that there isn't.

"With the lack of current evidence, we find it difficult to recommend mothers with well-controlled gestational diabetes to give birth in obstetric led unit with continuous fetal monitoring and deny them a chance to have home birth or birth in midwifery-led birth units." (Jabak & Hameed 2020)

Pain relief and other drugs in labour

Some of what there is to say about pain relief in labour if you have a higher BMI has already been discussed in the section on anaesthetic consultations in chapter five, and I will cover the use of birth pools and baths in more depth in the next section. But there are a couple of other things I want to add. It is worth thinking ahead about whether you might want pain relief in labour and, if so, what you might want to use. Women with a higher BMI are unfortunately more likely to experience pressure to use (or sometimes to not use) certain kinds of pain relief, and they may also come under pressure in other ways, so preparation for labour can be even more important than for women with a lower BMI. The points I am raising in this section are simply those relating to having a higher BMI. I wholeheartedly recommend that you do some general research as well, and perhaps look for an independent childbirth educator who will help you and your birth partner(s) learn about the options.

Some plus size women are advised to accept an epidural in early labour 'just in case' they need a caesarean. This is always your decision, of course, but there are pros and cons to epidurals and you may want to consider beforehand how you will respond to this offer and how your birth partner(s) can support you in this.

If you weigh more than average, then opiate drugs like pethidine (Demerol®) may not work as well for you. This is one situation where weight matters more than BMI. You may wish to discuss this with your midwife or doctor, who may be able to give you a slightly higher dose, although there is a limit to how much they can give you because this type of drug is known to affect babies, especially when given near birth.

Women with a higher BMI are sometimes offered a type of medication such as omeprazole during labour. This is called a proton pump inhibitor, and it usually comes in the form of a tablet. It reduces the acidity in your stomach and it is given just in case you need a caesarean. This isn't recommended in national guidance, but a number of midwives and women have told me it happens at a local level. Common side effects of omeprazole include headaches, feeling or being sick, stomach pain, flatulence (farting), diarrhoea and constipation. As with everything, it's your decision.

Finally, given the increased likelihood that larger women will be told they need intervention during labour and birth, I cannot overemphasise the value of staying active and mobile in labour, and in making sure you find or create an environment (in the widest sense of the word) that will help you labour well. If you are not giving birth in your own home, you may wish to stock a bag with things that you think might help you. These might include LED candles or fairy lights to help you create a relaxed atmosphere, personal comfort measures such as pillows, music, a birth ball, massage oil, essential oils, and anything else that you think might help you, such as a portable Bluetooth speaker for playing music.

Your caregivers may well seem to focus more of their time on the supposed risks of having a higher BMI, but there are lots of things that you can do in labour to give yourself the best chance of having a straightforward birth, and I would encourage you to focus your energy on this, as it can make all the difference to your experience. Another incredibly valuable form of pain relief, which also helps in many other ways, is to use a birth pool or bath in labour, so let's look at that next.

Using a birth pool or bath in labour

We have evidence from research into tens of thousands of births that using water for labour and birth is safe for both mother and baby, and that it leads to good outcomes with fewer interventions (Lukasse *et al* 2014, Henderson *et al* 2014, Cluett *et al* 2018, Ulfsdottir *et al* 2018, Maude & Kim 2020, Aughey *et al* 2021, Lanier *et al* 2021, Burns *et al* 2022). These and other studies show that water immersion significantly reduces maternal pain and thus the need for other kinds of pain relief, including epidural and opiates. It also decreases the chance of episiotomy and postpartum haemorrhage, increases the chance of an intact perineum and leaves women feeling more satisfied after birth (Burns *et al* 2022).

Water can aid buoyancy and mobility in labour (Benfield *et al* 2010), which can be particularly advantageous for some plus size women. Many of us are just as capable of moving around as women with a lower BMI, and sometimes more so.

Yet we know from research (Aughey *et al* 2021) and real-life experience that women with a BMI over 30 kg/m^2 are less likely to use a birth pool in labour in the UK than women with a BMI lower than 30 kg/m^2. Some studies of waterbirth (including Aughey *et al* 2021) have excluded women with a BMI over 35 or 40 kg/m^2, which means it's hard to get good data on whether the benefits may be similar or further increased in women with a higher BMI. In Burns *et al*'s (2022) review and meta-analysis *"only eight studies (22%) provided birth pool eligibility criteria regarding raised BMI. These studies did not include BMI as a characteristic in their analysis for interventions or outcomes. However, their inclusion in the study populations suggest that water immersion is not considered to be harmful for women who have raised BMI but are otherwise healthy."*

Unfortunately, women with a higher BMI (usually over 35 kg/m^2 or 40 kg/m^2, depending on the local guideline) are often discouraged or told they are 'not allowed' to birth in midwifery-led settings (NICE 2022), where the use of water pools is more prevalent. Women giving birth in hospitals may also be told that they may not use a bath or water pool. The reason given is usually to do with concerns about getting the woman out of the pool during labour, if she was unable to climb out herself. Although lifting equipment should be available for use in an emergency in hospitals, this equipment may not be present in midwifery-led units, or there may be other technical reasons for concern. Midwives' employers are (rightly) expected to look after their wellbeing. So while denying access is not equitable, it is often based on concerns about risk and about staff wellbeing.

When one analyses the situation, however, preventing women with a higher BMI from using a pool isn't logical or evidence-based. This is another situation in which BMI isn't the most helpful measure. A very short woman with a BMI of 40 kg/m^2 can easily weigh less than a very tall woman with a BMI which falls into the range considered acceptable for birth pool use. For this reason, some units have a weight limit on pool use. This is just as frustrating, however. There are a number of other arguments that can be made, which I will outline in case you can use them in your conversations.

First, the vast majority of women do not pass out in a birthing pool. In fact, Consultant Midwife Julie Frohlich and I worked out the approximate chance of a woman feeling faint and needing help to get out of a birth pool, based on data from a large London hospital. It turns out that, over the past few years, this has happened in less than 1 in 1000 labours, based on all women, not just those who have a higher BMI. I have since compared data with several other senior midwives, with similar results. None of us are aware of any incident of a woman with a higher BMI having collapsed in a birth pool. One might think, from listening to people talk about this risk, that women with a high BMI are going around regularly fainting in birth pools like Jane Austen heroines. In fact, larger women may even be less likely to do this than women with a 'normal' or low BMI, because of the obesity paradox and our increased blood volume and other reserves.

We also need to remember that labouring women are sane, intelligent people who do not wish to faint in a water pool any more than their caregivers wish for them to do so. In my experience, all midwives caring for women in birth pools in labour are vigilant for signs that a woman is feeling woozy, and will have a low threshold for asking her to step out of the pool, even temporarily, if they are concerned. In my experience, women who feel dizzy or faint in a birth pool will tell someone straight away and will often start to get out before they feel worse. If you are planning to use a pool and your caregiver is worried, you may wish to explain that you understand the risks, and will have a very low threshold for getting out of the pool if you feel even slightly lightheaded. You can also assure caregivers that you are aware of the need to keep well hydrated and nourished while you are in the pool, to empty your bladder regularly, and to maintain (and perhaps ask birth partners to maintain) an awareness of whether you are getting too hot. In countries such as the UK, guidance requires that midwives check the pool temperature and (with consent) the woman's temperature every hour, so this provides additional reassurance.

The next argument that women hear tends to be around the issue of excessive bleeding after birth. This is where it can be useful to remember the existence of the obesity paradox, in which larger women have more reserves to draw upon. This is a particularly relevant point if care providers are concerned about getting you out of a birth pool should you bleed excessively after birth. Larger women have a higher blood volume going into labour, as I will discuss again later in this chapter, which means that we can lose more blood before being compromised. This greater reserve means that we have a longer time period to get out of a pool before we are in danger of compromise.

In the very unlikely event that you do feel faint or bleed in a pool, there are still a number of other things that can be done. I realise that not everybody has a partner, and that not all partners are physically strong, but if you do have a partner who is physically strong, you can point out that they are unlikely to just stand by and watch you faint. Frankly, even if your partner isn't strong to begin with, it's amazing what a bit of adrenaline can do to one's ability if someone we love needs help.

It does seem counter-intuitive that lifting equipment is deemed to be so critical to some hospitals that they can't let you access something that is proven to be beneficial without it, and yet not critical enough that they will just buy the right equipment. In the 2010 version of the CMACE/RCOG guidance on '*Management of women with obesity in pregnancy,*' there was a recommendation that all maternity units should have safe lifting equipment that could lift up to 250kg (Modder & Fitzsimons 2010). However, the maximum weight part of this was omitted when the guidance was updated by Denison *et al* in 2018. But it is also possible to use other types of equipment to help women out of pools. Depending on the type and location of the pool, women may be able to roll across onto a bed, or be helped to use plastic steps. *"We have to adapt and innovate and manage when it's a so-called normal sized woman,"* one midwife told me. *"Why is it any different when someone's bigger?"* (Lou)

It is indeed true that midwives may not be able to lift you out of a pool, but the majority of midwives probably couldn't lift an eight stone (50kg) woman out of a pool without help, and if they need help or equipment to help a woman with a lower BMI then why can't the same equipment be used for women with a higher BMI? I am again not underplaying the fact that we need to protect midwives from injury, but other things that can be done include draining the water or, in the extremely unlikely event that every other idea fails, someone can support your head above the water while further help is called. This situation is so unlikely, however, that none of the practitioners I spoke to while writing this book, who have between them spent many years working in hospitals and birthing units which see tens of thousands of births each year, had even heard of this having ever happened. In the very small number of cases that people knew of where plus size women needed to get out of a pool quickly, this happened safely and successfully.

A couple of questions that I like to suggest that women ask during any conversations you might have about this, ideally in as innocent a voice as you can muster, are (a) what would happen if you fainted onto the bathroom floor during a land labour (because you would have to be helped up in that situation too), and (b) what happens if a woman with a lower BMI faints in the birth pool, and you're unable to lift her? These are interesting questions to ask because you will often find that, when you are given the answer, there's no reason that the same thing couldn't be done for you.

"Getting anybody out of the bath if they're unconscious and a dead weight is a challenge. It doesn't matter if they have a high BMI or not. It's just an excuse, it's about following the system." (Zoe, midwife)

Sometimes, hospitals or birth centres ask larger women to 'prove' that they can get in and out of the birth pool, by demonstrating this to them in late pregnancy. This is really not okay, because women whose BMI is lower are not asked to prove that they can do this, and there is no direct correlation between BMI or weight and fitness or mobility, but some women are happy to do it because they see it as the fastest way to be 'allowed' to use the pool.

Finally, please be aware that you do not have a right to use a birth pool in a hospital or birth centre setting in any situation, no matter what your BMI, size or shape. For example, someone else might have got in first! The only way to be certain that you will have access to a birth pool in labour is to plan to stay at home for part or all of your labour and birth and hire or buy a birth pool to use in your house. If you do that, then by all means have a think about how you would get out of it in an emergency, but do remember that this is highly unlikely and that there are many benefits to using water in labour, for you and your baby. Not least of which is the fact that you're less likely to have interventions that can lead to you having more problems after the birth.

Intravenous access in labour

In some countries, it is recommended that larger women have an intravenous cannula sited in early labour. This is a needle put into someone's hand or arm in case they need to be given intravenous fluids (a drip) later in labour or in an emergency situation. In the UK guidance, Denison *et al* (2018) recommend that, *"Women with a BMI 40 kg/m² or greater should have venous access established early in labour and consideration should be given to the siting of a second cannula."*

This is a 'just in case' measure which, as with everything, you do not have to agree to unless you want to. The reasoning for this is that it can be a bit harder to put a drip into someone who is a bit larger, although a competent anaesthetist should be able to do this quickly, even in an emergency. Another aspect of the argument is that larger women are more likely to need a caesarean. But this is a good example of how the medicalisation of labour and birth can become a self-fulfilling prophecy for some. Having a cannula can inhibit movement and be a reminder that things may go wrong, and both of these can hinder your ability to relax, let go, and allow labour to progress. It's also not ideal to have a cannula if you want to use a pool in labour. It is possible to take measures to protect a cannula site if it is truly essential, as I have argued elsewhere (Wickham 2019a). But it can be hard to keep dry, it can inhibit your movement in the pool, and there is a chance of infection. It's possible that these things will interfere with your ability to labour, and may increase your chance of needing a caesarean. But we're all different, and some people might find having a cannula reassuring. It's your decision.

Labour progress

We have already seen how some of the myths about BMI and the alleged risks of living in a bigger body have been translated into guidelines and practices which mean that women with a higher BMI are more likely to experience interventions, including caesarean, and less likely to have a straightforward birth. This is frustrating and problematic, because there are significant advantages in trying to help women with a higher BMI to experience a straightforward physiological birth. As Kerrigan *et al* (2015) describe, supporting physiological birth can help reduce interventions *"such as induction and caesarean, which in themselves confer additional health risks for obese women such as wound infection and deep vein thrombosis."* Both induction and electronic fetal monitoring (which I will discuss in the next section) reduce the likelihood of vaginal birth. Many women with a higher BMI are also told that they need a hormone drip (Syntocinon® or Pitocin®) to speed up (augment) their labour, because their progress (as measured by regular vaginal examinations, the results of which are plotted onto charts called partograms) is deemed to be inadequate.

Many studies show that plus size are perfectly capable of labouring 'under their own steam' and successfully giving birth to healthy babies (Hollowell *et al* 2014, Clark-Ganheart *et al* 2015, Ellekjaer et al 2017, Rowe *et al* 2018, Dalbye *et al* 2021, Jevitt *et al* 2021). We also have evidence that, even in hospitals, a midwifery-led approach leads to better outcomes for plus size women than an obstetrician-led approach, which may also be called consultant care. For instance, women in the USA with a higher BMI who are cared for by midwives have fewer interventions than women cared for by obstetricians, but equally good outcomes for mothers and babies (Carlson *et al* 2017).

A key reason why healthy women – including those with a higher BMI – have better outcomes, less intervention and higher levels of satisfaction in less medicalised environments is because those who work in these environments tend to focus on optimising physiology, and working with the hormones of the female body. The female body is designed to give birth, and most women will do this very successfully without the need for intervention if they just have a bit of support, which is about having the right environment as much as anything. We know that labouring women need privacy, low levels of light and disturbance, and to feel that they can trust themselves and those around them (Odent 1994, Walsh 2012, Buckley 2015, Wickham 2022).

When women are supported and surrounded by people expressing belief in their ability rather than introducing doubt by talking about how they are at risk, or not progressing well, or that interventions may be needed, it is perhaps inevitable that they will make better progress and have better outcomes. Imagine warming up for a sporting event or some sort of activity that you haven't tried before. Do you think you will do well if you're in an exposed, semi-public place full of strangers who are getting in the way of your body being able to do its thing, shaming you for its size, and expressing doubt in your ability? How about if you were instead getting ready in a warm, safe, quiet place where the people around you are cheering you on, following your cues, and telling you that you're amazing and can do this? It's the same with birth.

Plus size women are often told about research which allegedly shows that they are less likely to progress well and that their labour may need to be augmented (Sebire *et al* 2001, Zhang *et al* 2007, Heslehurst *et al* 2008, Cedergren *et al* 2009, Kominiarek *et al* 2011, Hollowell *et al* 2014, Kerrigan *et al* 2015,

Ellekjaer *et al* 2017). But much of this research is flawed and based on unproven beliefs. Some claims (for instance Zhang *et al* 2007) stem from laboratory experiments with uterine tissue rather than the experiences of real women in labour.

Sadly, the obstetric literature often uses the phrase 'failure to progress', which is a really unhelpful term that makes it sound like a woman's body is somehow defective. Yet as we have discussed, this situation may be more about provider impatience. Some midwives turn this around and talk about 'failure to wait', which reflects their view that the real problem lies in restrictive obstetric guidelines, rather than in female physiology. But what is really going on? Are some larger women truly unable to labour well? Is it that they just aren't doing it within the timeframe set down by obstetric guidelines? Or is something else going on here? Again we must question whether the problems attributed by some health care providers to the bodies of larger women actually stem from the misconceptions, myths and weight stigma embedded in health care and the wider culture.

Whatever the cause, in both spontaneous and induced labours, diagnosing 'failure to progress' is the single biggest reason for women with a high BMI being told they need a caesarean. In some studies, so-called 'failure to progress' accounts for about three quarters of the in-labour caesareans performed on women with a higher BMI (Holloway *et al* 2014, Ellekjaer *et al* 2017). Importantly, Ellekjaer *et al* (2017) found that these caesareans aren't genuine emergencies, but are being done because clinicians are deciding that women's bodies aren't meeting the limits for labour progress set by guidelines. So what is the evidence here?

Labour progress: what's the evidence?

'Failure to progress' is a label that doesn't tell us anything in itself about a woman's body. It's a very arbitrary label that is based on charts and ideas that even obstetricians don't agree on, and not a physical thing that we can measure in the way we can measure blood pressure or height. The 'need' for augmentation or caesarean is also not generally determined by a hard measure, such as a woman's blood pressure reaching a certain threshold. These things are based on subjective decisions, which is why it is important to ask whether there really is evidence that larger women need more help progressing in labour, or whether our current approach to higher BMI and birth may again be at the root of the issue. It's not hard to imagine how one's ability to labour may be inhibited if people are exchanging doubtful looks and shaking their heads because you're not keeping up, or waving caesarean consent forms around.

I have long argued that some clinicians' pre-existing lack of faith in the ability of women with a higher BMI to labour is playing a significant part in the higher intervention and caesarean rates experienced by plus size women (Wickham 2009, 2014, 2017, 2019b). I had been a midwife for about a decade before I came across the idea that larger women weren't as good at labouring, and that our wombs apparently contract less efficiently than the wombs of women with a lower BMI (Zhang *et al* 2007). I was a bit surprised to read this, to be honest, because I hadn't noticed that in my practice. In fact, even when other studies repeated the claim, I still didn't see it in the women I was caring for.

When I looked for the evidence, I came across some of the studies that I listed above, but I wasn't convinced by those which claimed that larger women's wombs were ineffective. Most of the studies were carried out in hospital environments, and in situations where it was impossible to tell whether women with a higher BMI really were given a fair chance at labouring under their own steam. In other words, it was impossible to tell whether it was their bodies, care provider attitudes, inappropriate length of labour limits, the fact that hospital guidelines were being interpreted differently for larger women, or a combination of these factors that was the issue. As Edwards (2019) points out, where data come from women having hospital births and include induced labours, we can't be sure whether this also reflects physiological labour, or if the same pattern would be seen in women who give birth at home or in homelike environments.

It's also important to consider how and what is being measured. Ellekjaer *et al* (2017) compared the length of labour and the type of birth of women of different BMI categories. While they found that BMI had no significant effect on the length of labour, they realised that this may have been because plus size women were being told they needed a caesarean sooner than women with a lower BMI. Their analysis led them to conclude that this was unlikely to be the result of larger women experiencing more problems, but was more likely the result of a more cautious approach from health providers. Such an approach is a good example of how weight bias affects practice, outcomes and the experiences of women and families.

It's findings like these which beg the question of whether the idea that larger women are more likely to experience 'failure to progress' is a self-fulfilling prophecy. Hollowell *et al* (2014) showed that, while higher BMI women having their first baby experienced more augmentation than women with a lower BMI, there was no difference when it came to women with a higher BMI having a second or later baby. As Lead Midwife Emma Rose asks, *"does this mean that health care professionals are more likely to trust that the multiparous women with a higher BMI would birth vaginally again?"* If so, that's potentially good news for those having later babies, but it means we really need to focus on plus size first time mums.

Other studies have shown that when women were cared for in a respectful way, which focuses on supporting female physiology and creating an environment conducive to birth, they labour well (Clark-Ganheart *et al* 2015, Carlson *et al* 2017, Rowe *et al* 2018, Dalbye *et al* 2021, Jevitt *et al* 2021).

Studies which directly contradict the received obstetric view continue to be published. Hautakangas *et al* (2022), for example, found that the women with a BMI over 35 kg/m^2 in their study actually had stronger contractions, although they were still more likely to be told they needed a caesarean. And Østborg *et al* (2022) showed that increasing BMI was associated with a shorter duration of the pushing stage of labour, which led Booker (2022) to question the 'one-size-fits-all' approach that is currently used.

During my research for this book, several midwives told me the same thing from their own experience.

"Independent midwives have different outcomes from those seen in obstetric care. I don't see any difference in outcomes between larger women and so-called average sized women in my care. Size just isn't a factor for me. But it makes you wonder what's happening in the system. Is it the fat shaming? I think it's also to do with increasing interventions and surveillance due to body size, which we don't do as independent homebirth midwives. I'd love to see some research comparing outcomes for larger women in standard hospital care versus independent midwife care. Maybe the fact that I haven't seen different outcomes is because I don't change my care according to the size of the woman. My guess is that it would be a combination of the impact of 'shame' and additional interventions." (Rachel Reed, midwife)

"If we can sneak higher BMI women into the birth centre, we just don't see the problems. Even with first-timers, to be honest. It's about how you care for them. Tell them they're gorgeous and we believe in them, and they blossom, and do just as well as anyone else. I'm certain the problem in the [consultant] *unit isn't the women, it's the attitudes towards them."* (Graça, midwife)

"I had a midwife colleague who was a much larger woman and she used to actively ask to look after other large women and she had an amazing knack of helping them have straightforward births and good outcomes. You could see them visibly relax when she went into the room, as if they were thinking, 'here's someone who's going to understand me and not shame me.' We ought to do research on that. Is that a study? What happens to the outcomes when larger midwives look after larger women?" (Anne, midwife)

These are important questions. I also don't want to totally dismiss the possibility that women with a higher BMI might have slightly different labour patterns, because there is some evidence that this might be the case. Ellis *et al* (2019) found that the cervixes of women with a higher BMI were dilating from 4-6cm a bit more slowly than was usually seen in women with a lower BMI. But different isn't synonymous with pathological, and some obstetricians and others are calling for extra time and patience to be given to women with a higher BMI (Teale 2020, Booker 2022). Given the many negative consequences of both induction (Rydahl *et al* 2019, Dahlen *et al* 2021, Wickham 2021a, Haavaldsen *et al* 2023) and caesarean (Sandall *et al* 2018), a bit of patience (as long as there isn't an actual problem) would be beneficial whether or not the issue is physiology, overly restrictive guidelines, and/or care provider attitudes.

I'm going to give the last word here to Julie Frohlich, who has worked in home, hospital and midwifery-led unit settings, who summarises the current situation well.

"The UKMidSS data [Rowe *et al* 2018] *are very encouraging about women with BMIs between 35 and 40, who did extremely well. And I think the reason the women in the UKMidSS data set did extremely well is that nobody's putting the fear of God into them. Nobody's saying, 'we've got to monitor you continuously, we've got to put an epidural into you, we've got to monitor your baby because we're worried.' Women that labour in obstetric units have the fear of God put into them, so I think it's not really about BMI per se, I think it's really that women aren't relaxed so they don't labour well, they don't get the right hormone cocktail, they get a lot of adrenalin because they're worried, because they've been so frightened, because they've been labeled as a high risk pregnancy. So I think it's more to do with the environment that women with a higher BMI tend to be guided towards labouring in, and the ethos and atmosphere and the practices of an obstetric unit are just not conducive to straightforward vaginal birth. Women with a higher BMI who labour on our home from home midwifery-led unit, we don't see that. I don't think there's anything absolute about BMI and labour dystocia."* (Julie Frohlich)

The myth of the fat vagina

There's one rather unpleasant myth that relates to labour progress that I also need to debunk in this section. In late 2019, an obstetrician in Scotland made a rude, untrue, unevidenced and misogynistic comment during a BBC radio programme which immediately led to other obstetricians and the Royal College of Obstetricians and Gynaecologists in the UK speaking out to refute what he had said. His claim, which I am repeating here only for the sake of anyone who has come across it and believed it, was that one reason for an increase in the caesarean rate is that larger women have increased fat tissue in the birth canal. In other words, to use the horrible term coined by journalists, 'fat vaginas'.

His comment that supposed fat deposits in the birth canals of larger women meant that we are more likely to experience obstructed labour was immediately debunked by another obstetrician, Dr Virginia Beckett, in her role as spokeswoman for the Royal College of Obstetricians and Gynaecologists. Dr Beckett explained that obstructed labour has nothing to do with fat in or around the vagina.

The claim that there is such a thing as 'soft tissue dystocia' actually pre-dates the misogynistic radio comment by several years, however. As long ago as 1997, researchers speculated that, *"perhaps dystocia due to an increased deposition of soft tissues in the maternal pelvis may lead to the observed increase in the cesarean delivery rate"* (Crane *et al* 1997). This was a purely speculative comment, which was not evidence-based and has never been shown to have even the slightest basis in fact.

Since then, medical imaging studies have either not found additional fat in the vaginas of larger women (Barau *et al* 2006) or they did find a few more fat compartments in larger women, but found this was not clinically relevant (Wischnik *et al* 1992). In other words, it makes no difference.

The studies that I have discussed in this chapter on labour progress provide additional support for this not being an issue, which means there is an abundance of evidence that the theory is wrong. Having looked thoroughly at the evidence on this topic, I can confidently assure you that there is no such thing as a 'fat vagina'. It's an incorrect, misogynistic, obstetric myth that has no basis in evidence or real-world experience.

Sadly, this is not the only untrue obstetric theory of its kind. If you would like to read more about the history of this area along with a more in-depth common sense explanation of why it doesn't stand up to scrutiny, plus size birth activist Pamela Vireday (2010) wrote an excellent summary, which is still relevant today and is freely available online.

Electronic fetal heart monitoring in labour

Several of the guidelines describing the care that women with a higher BMI should receive include a recommendation that they should be offered electronic fetal heart monitoring (EFM, which is also known as cardiotocograph or CTG monitoring) in labour. As is often the case, the word 'offered' is used here to illustrate what should happen, and not what does happen. In reality, most women are told that this needs to happen and will accept it because the 'offer' is encased in fear and the false concern that their baby may not be okay if they decline it.

The exact nature and cut-off point of the recommendation varies, depending on where you live. As I have already noted, this kind of variation often highlights a lack of good evidence for something, and sometimes a lack of agreement about what to do about the lack of evidence. The recommendation is made at a national level in Australia (RANZCOG 2019), where women with a BMI over 40 kg/m^2 are specifically advised to have continuous CTG monitoring, and women with a BMI of 30-40 kg/m^2 are advised to have it if they also have another risk factor, for instance they are aged over 40, or are 41 weeks pregnant or over (Small 2023).

In other countries, national guidelines acknowledge the lack of evidence, yet EFM is still a reality for many women with a higher BMI. In the UK, for instance, the RCOG (Denison *et al* 2018) acknowledges that there is no evidence in this area and directs one to the NICE intrapartum guidance (NICE 2022), which doesn't give a recommendation either, but leaves it up to the clinician or local hospital trust. In reality, we know that women who have a higher BMI are often told they need EFM by doctors, despite this lack of evidence or national recommendation. Colleagues in the USA also report that it is highly unusual for women who have a higher BMI not to be advised to have continuous EFM in labour, despite conflicting advice and the already mentioned lack of evidence.

In fact, there is an astonishing lack of evidence that EFM is effective (Lewis 2013, Sartwelle & Johnston 2018, Small *et al* 2020, Clark 2022, Politi *et al* 2023, Small 2023). This isn't just in women who are healthy (or 'low risk') but also in women perceived to be at higher risk (Small *et al* 2020, Small 2023). These studies show that EFM leads to more intervention without making any positive difference in the wellbeing of babies. You'll know from the previous section that 'failure to progress' is the single biggest reason that larger women are told they need caesareans, but fetal distress, as diagnosed via EFM, is also significant here. EFM has significant other impacts on the woman's experience of labour. This is partly because we know that it is harder to monitor women who are larger (Brocato *et al* 2019), and this fact has knock-on effects which lead to a higher chance of more interventions.

Obstetrician Kirsten Small has summarised the evidence in this area:

"There might be an increase in the risk of intrapartum stillbirth, neonatal death, and hypoxic ischaemic encephalopathy for women with higher BMI, but the findings are not consistent across studies. The absolute difference in risks, even when you add all three outcomes together, is under one percent. It is likely that women with health conditions complicating their pregnancy contribute more to this increase than healthy larger women, but I simply can't find sources of evidence to sort that out reliably." (Small 2023)

In other words, just as I found when I analysed the evidence in chapter four, there may only be a marginal increase in the absolute risk of adverse outcomes, and this risk may be due to other health issues, and not shape or size. Small continues:

"Having established there is a marginal increase in risk (maybe), to make a difference at a population level to the uncommon issue of poor perinatal outcome for women with higher BMI, you would need a potently effective intervention. So, this brings us to the point where someone has now recommended intrapartum CTG monitoring. Is there evidence CTG monitoring is the potent tool that can reverse any increased risk?

"There is evidence to suggest CTG monitoring might be harmful for women with a higher BMI, and no evidence to speak of to know whether or not it could possibly improve outcomes for the baby. Guideline advice favouring CTG use for women of high BMI isn't built on a sound evidence base." (Small 2023)

I mentioned above that there are wider issues with the process of monitoring when it comes to women with a higher BMI. Both Small (2023) and Julie Frohlich discuss this, explaining that intermittent auscultation is preferable. Intermittent auscultation is when the midwife or birth attendant listens to the baby's heartbeat every five or fifteen minutes (depending on the stage of labour) with a portable handheld device called a Sonicaid. This is less intrusive and it doesn't lead to the problems that can stem from electronic fetal monitoring.

"One problem is that our guideline says that women with a BMI over 40 kg/m^2 should have continuous electronic fetal monitoring in labour, and we know that continuous EFM in labour can be trickier when you've got more padding. It can be harder to keep the signal, you get a lot of loss of contact. You can put a fetal scalp electrode onto the baby's head, but this means that many women have their mobility restricted by the monitoring.

"And then the focus of the midwife is on the monitoring, not on the wellbeing of the woman herself, it's on, 'can I keep that trace continuous?' And actually if you think about it logically, it's ridiculous. If you do intermittent auscultation, you're listening for a full minute, at least every 15 minutes in the first stage of labour and at least every five minutes in the second stage. Why isn't there

some compromise? If you've got some loss of contact, why is that such a bad thing? If you're monitoring for ten out of every fifteen minutes, then that's okay. But midwives view it as an absolute failure if they can't keep that line going on that trace for that entire labour. They restrict women's movements in order to get that sacrosanct trace, and it has no additional benefit." (Julie Frohlich)

In summary, there is no evidence to support the use of electronic fetal monitoring in labour for women with a higher BMI, and there is good reason to request that intermittent auscultation is used instead, especially if you are aiming for a physiological birth or wanting to avoid further intervention or restriction of movement.

VBAC

There are a few important things to know if you are a woman with a higher BMI who has already had a baby by caesarean and are wanting to have a VBAC, or vaginal birth after caesarean. The first is that a recent study showed that the babies born to women with a BMI of 35 kg/m^2 or more have comparable outcomes after planned VBAC as after planned repeat caesarean (Tzadikevitch-Geffen *et al* 2021). However, you may be told that, if you plan a VBAC, you have a higher chance of needing another caesarean than a women with a lower BMI. And this has been the finding of some studies, but there are caveats.

When I was researching this area I found it interesting that the three studies cited in the RCOG guidelines by Denison *et al* (2018), which are Durnwald *et al* (2004), Juhasz *et al* (2005) and Hibbard *et al* (2006), are all older and from the USA. But the same finding has been seen in more recent US studies (Rietveld *et al* 2017), and in research carried out in other countries, including India (Gupta *et al* 2014) and the UK (Mone *et al* 2014). The caveats are the same ones that I have been discussing throughout this book. Everything that I said about the obstetric approach to risk, birth, monitoring, and labour progress is just as relevant here. Women who opt for

VBAC will be advised to birth in hospital and accept the continuous EFM and arbitrary timeframes that we know are at least part of the reason why larger women have more chance of being told they need a caesarean.

Another thing to know is that, while obstetric guidelines advise practitioners to carefully discuss VBAC with women who have a higher BMI, which often leads to an overfocus on the risks of this option, I can find no evidence which shows that plus size women have a greater chance of problems because of their BMI. Yet it is likely that the obstetric approach to women with a higher BMI may well increase the chance of intervention. I can't find a study which shows how many unnecessary planned caesareans are being done in order to prevent the need for one in-labour caesarean, but it's safe to assume that this is a significant number.

As with every decision, you'll need to weigh up the pros and cons for your situation. Yes, you have a higher chance of being told you need a caesarean in labour than if your BMI was lower. And yes, in another utterly ironic turn, you may well be advised that you cannot access the kind of care and settings that would give you a higher chance of a successful VBAC. Yes, if you need an emergency caesarean in a hurry, there are implications in terms of anaesthesia, as explained in chapter five. The caesarean operation may also be more challenging for the surgeon. But a UK study showed that the actual chance of the situation that most obstetricians are worried about – uterine rupture – is 1 in 476 (Fitzpatrick *et al* 2012). We also know from the research by Hibbard *et al* (2006) that a woman with a higher BMI is no more likely to experience uterine rupture than a woman with a more average BMI. However, there is clear evidence that, no matter your BMI, agreeing to have oxytocin for induction or augmentation of labour if you have previously had a caesarean increases the chance of uterine rupture generally (Goer & Romano 2012, Al-Zirqi *et al* 2017, Wallstrom *et al* 2018, Zhang *et al* 2021), so you may want to avoid this.

The authors of an audit of the care of women with a BMI

of 30 kg/m^2 or over in the UK found that, although women with a higher BMI are less likely to opt for a VBAC, about 50% of the women who do will be successful (Relph *et al* 2021). Given that most of these births took place in obstetric units, where many women are facing the kind of BMI-focused maternity care which may not give them the best chance of experiencing physiological birth, this statistic is actually more impressive than it sounds. I cannot find any data showing what happens in the specific situation where women with a higher BMI opt for VBAC in midwifery-led settings, or where care was more tailored to their needs, but it would be interesting to see if the success rate was higher. Relph *et al* (2021) conclude that, "*VBAC ... should be supported for women who choose it.*"

When we add in the consequences of caesarean, and the greater risks of this for women with a higher BMI (which I discuss at the end of this chapter), it can be seen that VBAC is worth considering. If you decide to plan VBAC, the evidence discussed elsewhere in this book about the impact of environment and setting means you may want to consider where and with whom you will give birth, and how you can create an environment that will give you the best chance of a straightforward vaginal birth.

The birth of the placenta

The birth of the placenta is described in medical terms as the third stage of labour, and there are two main ways in which the placenta can be born. One is for the placenta to be born naturally, after a physiological birth. After your baby is born, you will feel your uterus tighten and then you will push out your placenta, usually within an hour. The other option is for the third stage of your labour to be medically or actively managed. In this situation, you will be given an injection of a drug which makes your uterus contract, the umbilical cord will be clamped and cut, and then the midwife or doctor will hold a hand over your lower abdomen to protect your uterus from moving, and then pull on the cord to deliver the placenta by controlled traction.

These days, almost all women who give birth in systems of maternity care are advised to have active management for the birth of their placenta. This is because research has shown that this can reduce excessive bleeding during and after the birth of the placenta, although the authors of the Cochrane review note that the quality of the evidence is low (Begley *et al* 2019). I have co-authored a book on this topic if you are interested in looking at the evidence and debates in more depth (Edwards & Wickham 2018).

One of the key things to understand here is that, while it's entirely your decision, the reality nowadays is that many women have one or more medical interventions in labour, and the majority of these interventions can predispose to women losing more blood during the birth of their placenta. This means that active management of the third stage is a necessary consequence of medical management of birth, and sometimes the only option. If you have had an oxytocin drip to induce or augment labour, for instance, a physiological third stage is negated by the fact that you've already been given the drug that's used to facilitate the birth of the placenta, and stopping it quickly can cause bleeding.

The guidance describing care for women with a higher BMI often states that larger women have an even greater chance of experiencing excessive bleeding, which is also known as postpartum haemorrhage, or PPH. This is one of the few recommendations for which the guideline writers state that there is high-level evidence (Denison *et al* 2018), but the evidence that they point to is the same evidence that Begley *et al* (2019), the authors of the Cochrane review on this topic, described as low quality.

It is certainly true that a good number of studies carried out in hospital settings have shown that women with a higher BMI have a greater chance of experiencing PPH than women with a lower BMI (Sebire *et al* 2001, Zhang *et al* 2007, Heslehurst *et al* 2008, Fyfe *et al* 2012, Polic *et al* 2022). This is commonly suggested to be a result of the theory of poorer uterine tone that I discussed (and questioned) earlier in this chapter (Zhang *et al* 2007, Driessen *et al* 2011, Blomberg 2011). Sebire *et al* (2001) also theorise that this may be because women with a higher BMI are more likely to have larger babies and thus larger placentas. But, as we did with some of the situations relating to risk in pregnancy, it's important to look at the actual numbers and the wider issues.

In Butwick *et al*'s (2019) study of more than two million hospital births in California, in which researchers specifically looked for an association between maternal BMI and PPH, excessive bleeding (more than 500mL) was experienced by:

2.4% of women (1 in 42) with a BMI of less than 18.5 kg/m^2.
2.8% of women (1 in 36) with a BMI of 18.5-24.9 kg/m^2.
3.1% of women (1 in 32) with a BMI of 25-29.9 kg/m^2.
3.3% of women (1 in 30) with a BMI of 30-34.9 kg/m^2.
3.3% of women (1 in 30) with a BMI of 35-39.9 kg/m^2.
3.5% of women (1 in 29) with a BMI of 40 kg/m^2 and over.

We can again see that the absolute increase in risk isn't nearly as significant as is sometimes implied. There are also a few confounding factors. Plus size women tend to experience more interventions that can lead or predispose to higher blood loss, including induction and augmentation, especially when they birth in hospital.

It's also of note that we give the same dose of Syntocinon® or Pitocin® to all women, regardless of weight. No-one seems to have considered this as an issue, even though we know that larger people can sometimes need a higher dose for a medicine to be effective.

Another important consideration with most of the research studies in this area is that researchers measure blood volume that is lost and use this to decide whether or not someone had a PPH. Notwithstanding the fact that we know that our attempts to measure blood loss are notoriously inaccurate, we know that larger people have more blood to begin with. So it might actually be normal and expected for a woman with a higher BMI to lose a bit more blood than someone who is very light or slim. In fact, as I will come back to later in this chapter, this protective effect is one of the advantages of having a higher BMI, and is mentioned in at least one national PPH strategy document (OBS Cymru 2017). So the finding that larger women may, on average, lose more blood in terms of volume may not be as significant in reality as these findings make it sound on paper.

However, both the Birthplace study (Hollowell *et al* 2014) and the UKMidSS data set (Rowe *et al* 2018) found that women with a higher BMI didn't have higher rates of serious bleeding or blood transfusion in midwifery-led settings. In fact, Rowe *et al* (2018) found that multiparous women with a BMI of 35 kg/m^2 or higher were actually less likely to have a PPH of 1500ml than multiparous women with a lower BMI. This may be another situation where the way that people are treated and the monitoring and interventions that they are exposed to may have a greater effect than their BMI.

It is worth noting that most of the women in the Hollowell *et al* (2014) study had active management. In fact, the high number of women who have active management in general means that, although there is clear room for improvement in the quality of the research, it's hard to collect data on what would happen during a physiological placental birth. But I can't find any evidence to support the idea that a woman with a higher BMI who is healthy, has experienced a physiological labour and birth of her baby, and is wishing to have a physiological birth of her placenta would have a higher chance of experiencing a compromising blood loss than a woman who has a lower BMI. There are other factors that may be important, but it's hard to see how BMI would make a difference.

The complexities and uncertainties in this area mean we are left with more questions than answers. If researchers could (a) move away from a medicalised approach, (b) accept that medicalised birth is itself a significant risk factor for PPH, and may be more important than BMI, especially in hospital settings, and (c) take into account the fact that larger people have more blood in the first place, we could probably learn a lot more.

Caesarean section considerations

I have already discussed the fact that women with a higher BMI are more likely than women with a lower BMI to be told they need a caesarean, no matter whether their labour begins spontaneously or after induction (Bergholt *et al* 2007, Zhang *et al* 2007, Kominiarek *et al* 2010, Fyfe *et al* 2012, Crequit *et al* 2020, Dalbye *et al* 2020). However, this may well be partly or wholly the result of the guidelines and recommendations that exist around the care of women with a higher BMI in labour.

There is a curious paradox here. It is well accepted that larger people experience more risk during and after surgery of any kind, which is partly why there is a recommendation that women with a BMI of 40 kg/m^2 or higher meet with an anaesthetist in case surgery becomes necessary (see chapter five). Yet the abundant evidence about the low-tech, lower cost things that can reduce a woman's need for caesarean - such as midwife-led care, labour companionship, and the use of water for labour (Betrán *et al* 2018, Burns *et al* 2022) - is being ignored in favour of interventions that are actually more likely to result in surgical birth.

We also know that larger women are often encouraged to plan a caesarean rather than 'take the risk' of needing an emergency caesarean (Denison *et al* 2018). This is partly because different equipment may be required for women who have a very high BMI, but this equipment should be available in all hospitals and women should not be expected to take on risk because of health services' lack of planning. It is really questionable to be recommending a surgical procedure known to carry risks to a healthy woman who is capable of giving birth physiologically, who wants to give birth physiologically, and who has a good chance of being able to give birth physiologically if only her care providers would support her to do that rather than introducing fear and doubt at every turn.

That said, some women with a higher BMI do need or want caesareans, and there are a few things that need to be considered. One is that larger women have a higher chance of wound infections after having a caesarean (Sebire *et al* 2001), so antibiotics are strongly recommended (Denison *et al* 2018, Neal & Teale 2019). However, antibiotics are recommended as an intrinsic part of surgery for all women, regardless of BMI. The chance of experiencing VTE is increased if someone has a caesarean, so measures will be taken during and after the surgery to reduce this risk. These may include special inflatable devices on your legs during and after the surgery, and blood thinning drugs. I look at these and other postnatal (after birth) issues in the next chapter.

Over the years, there have been some debates amongst obstetricians about surgical techniques, including which kind of incision (cut) is the best to use, whether or not to use a drain, what is the best repair technique, and what is the best surgical dressing to use. There isn't clear evidence favouring one approach over another, and I don't have space to go into the nuances of this debate here. Vireday (2017a) wrote a helpful and freely available overview of the debate on surgical techniques if you would like to explore it in more depth. There is also variation depending on where you live, so this is best discussed with your own midwife or obstetrician. I will mention that some surgeons are more likely to use staples to close the wound when a woman with a higher BMI has a caesarean. The use of staples means that you are likely to need an additional postnatal appointment to have these removed.

There are some helpful resources, books, and people out there if you want to know more about caesareans generally. The most important thing to know is that if you are offered a caesarean it is always good to ask lots of questions, including what your options are. This is a crucial decision, because agreeing to surgery will have implications for you, your baby, and any future pregnancies and births.

The advantages of higher BMI in birth

There are some advantages to having a higher BMI during labour and birth, and some things that plus sized women are at less risk of. I think it's just as important to highlight these as it is to discuss the risks associated with being larger. Sadly, most of the writers of obstetric guidelines don't agree with me, and they focus solely on discussing supposed risks, not all of which are supported by evidence.

I mentioned above that multiparous women with a BMI of 35 kg/m^2 are less likely to have significant bleeding after birth than women with a lower BMI (Rowe *et al* 2018), and that all plus size women have another advantage when it comes to blood loss at birth, in that they have a higher blood volume (OBS Cymru 2017). A similar large blood loss will thus be far more impactful on a smaller woman than a larger woman, because women with a higher BMI have this higher reserve of blood. As another example of the obesity paradox, this may partly explain why larger people are more likely to survive some diseases than those with a lower BMI. In simple terms, we have more reserves for our bodies to draw upon when receiving treatment and recovering.

Some independent midwives that I have worked with and spoken to think that larger women may cope better with longer labours, which may also be about having better reserves. Rachel Reed describes how *"as a midwife, I'm more worried about the slim, not well-nourished women. There's something to be said for some fat stores."* This may be one reason why plus size women do better in midwifery-led settings, where their physiology and individuality is respected.

Another advantage was postulated by Gurol-Urganci *et al* (2013), who suggested that women with a higher BMI may be less likely to have an obstetric anal sphincter injury (OASI or OASIS). This is a tear that extends to or involves the muscle that controls the anus, often called a third or fourth degree tear. I have become aware from colleagues over the years that audit data from several hospitals also shows that women with a higher BMI have fewer serious tears. Audit data is not always published publicly, but it is sometimes presented at conferences. Julie Frohlich has identified a protective effect of higher BMI on third degree tear rates in audit data from a large London hospital. Those data show that 43% of OASIs happen in women with a BMI of up to 22 kg/m^2 and 29% occur in women with a BMI of 22-25 kg/m^2. So 72% of the OASIs in that audit happened in women with a BMI of 25 kg/m^2 or less.

An Australian study also showed that women with a BMI of 25 kg/m^2 or more were significantly less likely to have an OASI than women whose BMI was less than 25 kg/m^2. The protective effect of high BMI against OASI was even greater for the women who had a BMI of more than 35 kg/m^2 (Constable *et al* 2020).

These topics aren't being researched nearly enough. When they are accidentally discovered, the findings are often not highlighted. This reflects something called publication bias, and it's partly linked to the fact that the current medical and cultural viewpoint on BMI are very pervasive. Findings showing that larger people have any kind of advantage would (and do) cast doubt upon the current viewpoint. They provide an argument against weight bias, and could cause people to question other ideas. In the eyes of someone like myself, that would be a very good thing, as it can lead to a more nuanced understanding and perhaps a better approach. In the eyes of those who profit from having people think that they're at risk, this doesn't align with their goals, so the data aren't shared. I realise that this may sound cynical, but I think it's an important point to mention.

There may well be other advantages to being larger, but until more of us go looking for them and also create spaces where they can be discussed, we won't see them in the medical or mass media.

Tips for labour and birth

Many of the tips that I offered at the end of chapter five are also relevant during labour and birth, and there are a few additional things you might want to consider.

Think ahead about where you want to labour and give birth and what you might want in order to create the environment that is right for you. The data clearly show that plus size women are more likely to be told they need intervention in labour, which means that it is well worth thinking about (a) how you will respond to offers of intervention and (b) whether there are positive things you can do to prepare ahead of time.

If there are things that you particularly want in labour, such as the use of a birth pool, then look into that as early as possible. See the tips at the end of chapter five for more.

You may want to write a birth plan which clearly states your wishes, and ensures that anyone looking after you in labour is aware of this.

It can also be important to think about who you might want to have with you, and whether that person or those people will advocate for you if you need that. This might be family members, friends, trusted professionals, or hired birth workers. Are these people size friendly? If not, do you really want them in your birth space? This isn't the time to be nice!

Some women who wish to avoid non-essential birth interventions spend time in pregnancy gathering and bookmarking information which they can refer back to if something is offered in labour, when they are more tired. It is not up to you to prove anything to a health professional, but some people have found it beneficial to be able to point doctors towards the evidence, or to have their partner do that.

As you are thinking through these issues and questions, you might find it helpful to gather more information from books. *What's Right For Me?* can help you think ahead about birth-related decisions (Wickham 2022), or see *In Your Own Time* for more on induction (Wickham 2021a). This is where antenatal groups, classes, or other educational resources can come in really handy too.

As with the tips at the end of the pregnancy section, if you don't know who will be looking after you in labour ahead of time, you may wish to tell your caregiver at the outset that you don't want to discuss your weight or have a particular intervention. A useful statement is, *"I'm aware that you may be obliged to raise the question of BMI or [intervention X], but I have looked at the evidence and have decided I don't want that."*

It can be useful to women of any size or shape to think about mobility in labour. How flexible you are and how easily you are able to get into different positions is not about size, shape, or weight. I mention this because the way that larger women are sometimes treated by health professionals means that we may benefit from measures which promote mobility and physiology even more than women with a low or average BMI. Are there things you would like to have around you in labour to help with that? Some examples of things that can help mobility include a water pool, a step to help you in and out of the pool, a birth ball, and beanbags and pillows to help you get into different positions. I will return to this in my tips for after the birth as well, but if you decide to have a hospital birth then you may wish to take extra pillows for comfort if you need or decide to stay in hospital after the birth.

The following list won't be for everyone, but a wrap skirt has helped several women feel less exposed when pushing, if they agreed to being examined, or when giving birth in a hospital setting. Comfort measures such as wet wipes can be great if you tend to sweat (no matter what your size). It is also worth thinking about what kinds of bras, underwear and tops will be most comfortable for you. Shawls, big scarves, wraps or rebozos can help with privacy, especially in a hospital. I will explain this further in the next chapter but it may also be worth investing in a pair of surgical stockings that fit you well and are the right size, and putting these in your labour bag if you plan a hospital birth or agree to transfer to hospital in labour.

7. After the birth

When I was writing this book, one of the most common things I heard women and midwives saying in relation to the postnatal period went something like this:

"It makes me so sad to live in a world where apparently the most important thing is to 'get your body back' after giving birth. We should be focusing on mental health and take a more holistic approach to helping women with new babies." (Marianna, doula)

Ideally, everyone would have lots of people around them to support them in their transition to becoming parents, to give any assistance they need with recovery, and to help with things like house and garden work while they adapt to their new situation. In reality, many women find that they lack support and have difficulties adapting, and women with a higher BMI face some additional pressures.

Recovering from birth

Although birth is a physiologically normal experience that the female body is well designed to undertake, it can also be physically and emotionally tiring, and it's totally normal to need some recovery time. In fact, it's advantageous to take time away from your everyday life to get to know your new baby, to establish feeding, and to explore the new ways of being, doing and living that come with having a new tiny person (or people) in your life.

Recovery will look different for everyone and it is my experience as a midwife that health, fitness, type of birth, support, and how you experienced the last few weeks of pregnancy are much better predictors of how you'll cope after the birth than your BMI or weight. I truly think that the most important thing that everyone can do after birth is to listen to their body and follow its cues. But there are a few situations in which you might need or be offered additional interventions if you have a higher BMI during the postnatal period. Some of these, including dietary interventions and injections to reduce the chance of thromboembolism, are offered both before and after birth, so I won't repeat everything that I wrote in chapter five. I'm just going to add extra information or statistics here that relate to the postnatal period, so please see chapter five if you need a reminder about why these are offered, or what the side effects might be.

Postnatal weight loss advice

The postnatal period is often seen as a good time to give weight loss advice. As Pamela Vireday (2017b) summarised:

"There is intense pressure from some care providers to lose pregnancy weight gain after the baby is born. This is because many women do retain weight from pregnancy long-term and never go back to their pre-pregnancy weight, resulting in a permanent net gain. However, the best way to return to pre-pregnancy weight is hotly debated."

Given what the literature on dieting shows about how ineffective this is for most people in the longer term, I would add that there are also questions not only about how this is possible, but also about whether it is possible for everybody. Nonetheless, the pressure to lose weight after a baby is born is further evidenced by the number of studies which test diets and call for more action in the area of postnatal weight loss (Bick *et al* 2020, Lim *et al* 2022, Liu *et al* 2022). Pressure is put on women to attend classes, heed weight loss advice and go on diets.

It is concerning that so little consideration is given to the already significant pressures that women and families are experiencing in the days and weeks after a baby is born. Social support is lacking for new parents, who are also struggling with sleep, an ongoing reduction in postnatal care, and facing a significant learning curve as they learn to care for their new arrival. Many parents prioritise the needs of their baby, other children, and family members over their own. They may not have time to follow special diets or plan, shop for, prepare and cook the suggested diet plans, not to mention the current cost of living crisis affecting so many families. Few studies on this topic acknowledge the reality of life as a new parent, and I haven't seen this mentioned in any guideline.

A good portion of the research on postnatal weight loss is funded by the diet industry. This may not always be apparent in the papers. I found several studies where funded members of slimming organisations were involved, but their conflict of interest was not disclosed, sometimes because they were not among the lead authors. Many of the studies on postnatal weight loss are poorly designed (or perhaps they are well designed, if the intention was to show the results that support the status quo, rather than looking for the truth about whether dieting benefits new mothers). For example, participants may be self-selected, the intervention and control groups are not always comparable, and those who took part aren't followed up for long enough to show what happened to their weight or BMI in the medium or long term.

The better designed studies tend to find that postnatal weight loss programmes are either not effective (Vinter *et al* 2014) or that women can lose weight in the short term, but will regain it a few months later (Ronnberg *et al* 2016). There is also some evidence that an intuitive eating approach (which avoids weighing, measuring, recording and assessing dietary intake) can be more beneficial, although this was based on retrospectively asking women what had worked for them, rather than a trial to test such an approach (Leahy *et al* 2017). Some studies state that the most effective form of postnatal weight loss is breastfeeding (Vinter *et al* 2014), but this isn't straightforward either. And, ironically, larger women are not always given the support they need to help them breastfeed. I will discuss both these issues later in this chapter.

Wound healing

One of the things that we have good evidence on is that plus size women who have had a caesarean are more likely to get a surgical site infection than women with a lower BMI (Wloch *et al* 2012, Saeed *et al* 2017). This can occur in up to 15% of women (Saeed *et al* 2017). So the prevention of infection is a key focus of recommendations, which includes giving antibiotics during caesareans (Denison *et al* 2018). It's not hard to work out why wound infections are more likely if you have a bigger body. Wounds heal faster when they are dry, clean and exposed to air. If you have a bigger tummy, then your caesarean wound isn't going to get as much air as if you had a lower BMI, and the area is likely to be warmer, moist, and thus more prone to bacterial growth. For that reason, it's important to wash daily, with just water, and then gently pat yourself dry.

I'm not convinced that all plus size women are given appropriate information about the simple everyday things they can do to help themselves here, though. So I'm going to spell it out. In any situation where someone has a wound, careful and consistent hygiene can do marvels. You will probably have a dressing on for a few days but, once that has come off, make sure you take time to dry thoroughly after a shower or bath. If the house is warm enough, lying on your bed and exposing your wound to air can be a really good way of ensuring that it really is dry before you get dressed again. Get comfy, move your tummy out of the way, and use pillows or rolled up towels to support yourself so you're not straining muscles. Allow someone to help you if you need it, and remember that this isn't an exercise in elegance.

It can also be useful to deliberately expose your wound to air at other times. This will help ensure that the area around it is not going to be wet, warm and creating an environment in which bacteria can flourish. As midwife and lactation consultant Katie James explains, this can have the dual benefit of helping you to rest and helping with breastfeeding.

"Use [it] *as an excuse to have a 15 minute lie down with your knickers round your ankles. Lie on a towel, and add in an extra bit of skin to skin with your baby, several times a day."* (Katie James)

It is also really important to rest as much as possible, to not be moving about so much that you're getting overheated (although you do want to be moving a bit - we'll get to that), and to pay attention to how your wound is healing. Many women (no matter their size or shape) can't see their wound themselves, so you can ask someone else to look, or use your phone to take a picture. If you're concerned, or think your wound doesn't look right, talk to your midwife as soon as possible.

I have a bit more to say about wound healing in relation to breastfeeding, so please see that section too.

Back to VTE and heparin

One of the most significant interventions offered to some women with a higher BMI in the postnatal period are the low molecular weight heparin (LMWH) injections that I began to discuss in chapter five. I want to mention again at the outset that a small subset of women have a very high chance of a type of blood clot called venous thromboembolism (VTE). This includes anyone who has experienced a previous VTE, has a blood clotting condition, or who is very immobile after birth. The issues discussed in this section don't relate to those who are at very high risk, but to the women who are offered heparin in the postnatal period because they have one or more common risk factors, which includes higher BMI.

I've already mentioned in chapters four and five that the chance of experiencing VTE is a bit higher for women of any BMI in the postnatal period than during pregnancy (Butwick *et al* 2019). There are a number of reasons for this. Women's bodies have lost some blood and fluid, which is normal and healthy, but this can increase the chance of a blood clot developing. We are likely to be a bit more sedentary after giving birth, not least because it's tiring. We tend to sit or lie down a bit more to regather our energy after birth and to feed and cuddle our babies. Caesarean surgery and some other medications and interventions can also increase the chance of VTE. On an individual basis, the data show that the absolute risk of experiencing VTE is still very low after birth, but there is an increased chance of VTE after birth when we look at population-level data. As a reminder, Butwick *et al* (2019) found that, after birth, VTE was experienced by:

2.0 in 10,000 (1 in 5000) women with BMI up to 18.4 kg/m^2.
3.1 in 10,000 (1 in 3226) women with BMI of 18.5-24.9 kg/m^2.
3.9 in 10,000 (1 in 2564) women with BMI of 25-29.9 kg/m^2.
5.6 in 10,000 (1 in 1786) women with BMI of 30-34.9 kg/m^2.
9.0 in 10,000 (1 in 1111) women with BMI of 35-39.9 kg/m^2.
13.2 in 10,000 (1 in 758) women with BMI 40 kg/m^2 or more.

There is some variation between countries as to who will be offered heparin after birth. In the UK, for example, any woman with a BMI of 40 kg/m^2 or more is likely to be offered these injections for ten days after birth, even if she doesn't have other risk factors. The same is true for any woman who had an unplanned caesarean, regardless of BMI. Then, anyone with two or more risk factors from another list may be offered heparin, sometimes for a longer period of up to a few weeks.

The table of risk factors can easily be looked up online and it includes having a BMI over 30 kg/m^2, being 35 or older, having had a planned caesarean, a PPH of more than 1000ml, twins or more, preterm birth, prolonged labour, and stillbirth, along with several others (RCOG 2015, Denison *et al* 2018). As some of these risk factors are to do with things that happen during labour and birth, and as one doesn't need to have many risk factors to be deemed to be 'at high risk' in the postnatal period, a considerable number of women with a higher BMI are offered heparin after birth.

We know from midwives, doctors, women, and published papers that a sizeable proportion of women decide not to take these injections (Teale 2020). In one study, about a third of women opted not to give themselves the injections as they had been directed to (Rottenstreich *et al* 2020). It may be that the actual figure is even higher, as some women take the injections home but elect not to tell their midwife or doctor that they are not injecting themselves with the heparin.

There is concern about the downsides of this intervention, as well as the data on which its use is based. As I explained in chapter five, obstetricians in most countries don't see any benefit to offering heparin in pregnancy (ACOG 2018), and even those who offer it after birth acknowledge the lack of evidence of benefit for heparin in women with common risk factors, along with the fact that the risk screening tools that are used have not been validated by research (ACOG 2018, Kotaska 2018, 2021).

The authors of the Cochrane review *'Preventing venous thromboembolism in women during pregnancy, childbirth and after birth'* concluded: *"The evidence is very uncertain about benefits and harms of VTE thromboprophylaxis in women during pregnancy and the early postnatal period at increased risk of VTE."* (Middleton *et al* 2021)

Many women have the risk factors used to target offers of heparin, so large numbers of women are now being offered these injections in order to try and prevent something that occurs only rarely. A Canadian obstetrician, Andrew Kotaska (2018, 2021), has written a number of papers questioning this aspect of the way that heparin is being offered. He observes that *"the benefits of heparin are exaggerated and its harms are under-appreciated,"* and points out that we have no idea how many women need to be giving themselves heparin injections in order to prevent a single case of VTE (Kotaska 2018).

What we also know from Kotaska's (2021) analysis is that the specificity of these risk assessment tools in women with common risk factors (such as high BMI, older maternal age and caesarean birth) is low, at 0.13%. This means that only 0.13% of the women who are told they are at high risk for VTE after birth would experience a VTE, which is about 1 in 800. The chance is even lower during pregnancy, although we don't have exact figures on that.

Another important issue is that some of the prediction models which have been used in making decisions about offering heparin use data which could be misleading. Kotaska

(2021) explains that the studies used to provide the estimates of risk of VTE cited in guidelines used in the UK, Australia, Canada, Sweden, and New Zealand included asymptomatic VTEs. In other words, the researchers scanned healthy people who didn't all have symptoms of VTE, and looked to see if they could spot signs of possible blood clots. This means that the researchers identified and counted possible blood clots in the study that would have resolved themselves and wouldn't even have been known about if they hadn't been in the study. When statistics from such studies are used to support a recommendation of heparin, it can make it sound as if VTE is more common than it really is. This is why I shared data from the Butwick *et al* (2019) study, which looked at actual cases of VTE.

Kotaska (2018) also notes that previous editions of the guidelines in this area were written by panels including people who had *"financial and intellectual conflicts of interest."* These people have since been removed from the panels, but this doesn't necessarily eliminate their influence completely, because obstetric guidelines tend to be based on previous guidelines rather than created from scratch each time. It is also far more difficult to remove an intervention that has been adopted into use than it is to introduce one in the first place.

I want to share a bit more about why the UK has a more interventionist approach to VTE than other high-income countries, as I think this helps explain another aspect of the issue. In 2014, a report showed that VTE was the leading cause of maternal death and that this disproportionately affected some women with a higher BMI (Knight *et al* 2014). Between 2009 and 2011, 30 out of 252 maternal deaths in the UK were attributed to VTE, which is 1.26 per 100,000 maternities, or 1 in 79,365 maternities. Here, a 'maternity' means a pregnancy or birth experience, no matter how it ended. We have to count maternities rather than women in this kind of research, because quite a few women would have had more than one baby during that time period.

It is always tragic when anyone dies in or around birth,

and it is therefore important that we look at whether there are things we can do to reduce the chance of this in the future. But it is equally important that we consider all aspects of the situation, to make sure that any interventions introduced in the hope of preventing one set of problems are proportional and do not cause more problems in themselves. This is one of the concerns with heparin injections.

The potential harms of postnatal heparin after surgery in general include an increase in bleeding (Mismetti *et al* 2001, Zareba *et al* 2014), and in postnatal women this is linked with a higher chance of wound complications, which can result in re-hospitalisation (Ferres *et al* 2011, Lindqvist *et al* 2011). This is a particularly concerning finding given what I wrote above about plus size women having more chance of problems with wound healing in the first place.

A group of researchers in Alabama looked at the medical records of childbearing women before and after the policy of offering heparin to those deemed to be at risk was introduced. They found that, while women were more likely to receive heparin after the policy was introduced, there was no difference in the rate of VTE before and after its introduction. However, after heparin was brought in, women experienced significantly more wound haematomas (where blood pools in one area), more unplanned surgical procedures and more blood transfusions (Lu *et al* 2021).

Like Kotaska, the researchers concluded that *"guidelines recommending this strategy should be reconsidered"* (Lu *et al* 2021). I want to share a final quote from Kotaska's work on this, because I think it will help to explain how important it is to understand that, sometimes, the arguments made to support interventions are not logical. He wrote that:

"Proponents of liberal chemoprophylaxis [heparin] *claim that randomized trials are not feasible. Because the benefit of low-molecular-weight heparin is so small, the required sample size is enormous. At the same time, they claim that the risk of VTE is so great that widespread administration of low-molecular-weight heparin is justified without evidence. This is a nonsensical argu-*

ment: the risk cannot be simultaneously too small to measure and yet too great to make measurement unnecessary." (Kotaska 2021)

It is of course your decision whether or not to have heparin injections or not, before and after the birth of your baby, and you can now weigh up the evidence (where it exists) along with your individual situation in order to make the decision that is right for you.

As I discussed in chapter five, there are some other things you can do to reduce your chance of developing a blood clot. These include getting up and moving around frequently, keeping yourself well hydrated, taking care to move your legs and ankles often, and not crossing your legs while sitting. Compression socks can be helpful, but some larger women have found that hospital-provided socks are uncomfortable or not the right size. I know several plus size women who recommend buying your own if you can. Some women report being glad they had done this because the ones they were given in the hospital didn't fit properly. Others have told me that they felt embarrassment when a fuss was made by maternity support staff about getting the right size stockings for them, and they recommend bringing your own in order to avoid stress.

Breastfeeding

When it comes to breastfeeding there are some things that plus size women might want to be aware of, and some myths that need exposing. Let's start with the things that are clear. We have good evidence that women with a higher BMI are less likely to start and continue breastfeeding (Ramji *et al* 2018), which means that guidelines often recommend that extra support be given to women with a higher BMI who are wanting to breastfeed (Denison *et al* 2018). It is also important to know that many larger women do breastfeed successfully, and there is every reason to think that you can, too. The point of this section is to explain the issues so that, if you want to breastfeed, you can ensure you get the support and information you might need.

There are a few reasons why women with a higher BMI might be less likely to successfully breastfeed. While some researchers suggest that lactogenesis (or the production of breastmilk) can be a bit slower in larger women (Preusting *et al* 2017), it is also acknowledged that the cause of any delay is *"likely to be multifactorial in origin and may be due to women's perceptions of breastfeeding, difficulty with correct positioning of the baby and the possibility of an impaired prolactin response to suckling"* (Denison *et al* 2018).

We have seen throughout this book that plus size women are more likely to have interventions, such as caesareans and hormone drips to induce or speed up labour, and these can interfere with breastfeeding initiation. The weight stigma and bias experienced by many women with a higher BMI won't help either, as a midwife and lactation consultant explains:

"It's really hard to tease out the effects of labour and birth intervention on lactation physiology from the way we also care for larger women postpartum. They've maybe had a caesarean, an epidural, they may overhear midwives or doctors talking about them and the size of their bodies or the shape of their breasts, then in addition perhaps they're not getting enough or the right kind of support to feed their baby on the breast effectively ... For me, this is often a cascade, where one factor can lead to another and ends up resulting in early difficulties establishing milk supply or ineffective attachment to the breast. There are significant psychological aspects at play here, that may be long ingrained from society. And if you're being called names by your own healthcare provider and have had to deal with social stigmas for a long time, it is completely understandable that a woman may also find it very hard to breastfeed in public or show her breasts and body when she's on the ward or in the breastfeeding drop in clinic." (Katie James)

Just as with other aspects of the care of women with a higher BMI, the fact that it is difficult to separate the effects of physiology, weight stigma, and the psychological and social aspects of breastfeeding means that we need to be careful when making assertions that BMI alone is the problem. There's no evidence that this is the case. Research also shows that body image is an important factor. Brown *et al* (2015) and Hicks and Brown (2016) found that it was very common for new mums to worry about their postnatal body and about breastfeeding in public.

"Perhaps a bigger predictor [than BMI] *of whether a woman breastfeeds or not is her body image. How she feels about her body, regardless of weight, seems to be important. ... Mothers who are concerned about changes to their body shape, how pregnancy and birth affect their body and weight gain are less likely to plan to breastfeed. If they do breastfeed at birth, they only do so for a short period of time. Interestingly, this isn't anything to do with weight; body image issues affect those with a healthy BMI and even those who are underweight."* (Brown 2021: 207)

Midwives and lactation consultants who are working with breastfeeding mothers report spending a lot of time trying to undo the damage that has occurred as a result of myths, weight stigma, inaccurate depictions of breastfeeding, a lack of representation of a range of breast sizes and shapes in the media, and disrespectful care. For example:

"We hear people say that your breasts will suffocate baby. No, they won't, this should not be a barrier to trying out breastfeeding. Assumptions are made that larger breasts means large nipples which are too big for the baby's mouth! No, there's no correlation, some women with very small breasts have large nipples, and vice versa. Breastfeeding is harder? Well, it can be, but there are things you can do." (Katie James)

Plus size women are often told (sometimes with looks or gestures rather than words) that their shape or belly will get in the way, or that their breasts are too large, soft or pillowy. But, as Katie goes on to explain, we simply need to think about position, mobility and comfort. As several midwives mentioned to me the importance of taking particular care with positioning for women who have a higher BMI and want to breastfeed, I include the following explanation to illustrate how and why positioning can be a key source of problems, yet one that is also easily solved.

"Nearly all of us, larger or not, have some tummy left after birth,

it doesn't just disappear. If you've then got a breast that sits on top of your postpartum tummy, it may feel hard to find the room to position your baby to attach to the breast. Some people then lift up their breast to attach baby for a feed. However, the weight of the lifted breast will eventually want to go back to where it normally 'lives', and so it starts to fall out of the baby's mouth.

"With this two common things occur. Firstly as the breast tissue slides out of the baby's mouth the baby clings on to their milk supply at all costs, often meaning only the nipple is in the baby's mouth during the feed. Nipple feeding, i.e ineffective attachment, is when nipple pain, damage and cracks can occur.

"Secondly, as a result of the baby not being well attached, the milk cannot be removed effectively, leading to poor milk transfer, potential weight loss in the baby, as well as insufficient stimulation of the hormones of lactation needed to build and maintain an adequate milk supply for the future.

"The answer is to look for positions where women are more reclined, where you're not holding the baby in the standard textbook position. The baby doesn't have to be up high, like in the photos. It's likely to need to be a much more laid back, relaxed style. The baby might be sitting in your lap; that's a lovely, comfy position. But it's not a classic position, it's not the tummy to tummy picture that we see in the books. See where your nipples point and where your breasts are, how you can both feel comfortable and go from there!" (Katie James)

A few breastfeeding tips

The following tips are offered by a number of midwives, women and others who shared their experiences with me.

Do whatever you can to create a nest for you and your baby, set up what you need around you and maintain skin to skin as much as possible.

Use pillows to make your nest and to make yourself cosy and comfortable more generally. If you're planning to birth in hospital where the beds are small, take extra pillows with you to make it comfy. Put pillows under your arms if you're sat up and move them so you feel relaxed when you lie down.

Try to keep your baby with you (rather than in a cot, or with other people) as much as possible in the first hours and days after birth. This will help you recognise your baby's reflexes and cues and develop your own instincts. It will enable you and your baby to learn about each other.

Bear in mind that everyone's breasts are different, and the breastfeeding pictures and positions that you see in books, or are told about in groups, might not be the ones that work best for you. Read the tips on ergonomics in the next section, as they will help you understand more about what might help.

You may find it useful to look up Suzanne Colson's work on biological nurturing, or laid-back breastfeeding, if you're not already familiar with this (Colson 2019).

Some larger women or women with larger breasts find it helpful to put a rolled-up facecloth or small towel under their breast to change the position of their nipple, so you can see it.

There are also breast slings that you can buy, which clip onto your bra and hold your breast up. These don't work for everyone, but they can be helpful for some women.

Don't rely only on what the system is offering. It might not be enough, or it might not be size friendly. Gather phone numbers and find out about support, local experts, and drop in sessions in pregnancy.

Tips for midwives, birth workers and supporters

A few things are also consistently mentioned by those who are focused on offering appropriate, caring and respectful breastfeeding support to larger women, and many of these tips apply to caring for women at other times as well.

Individualised assessment is seen as vital.

"The most important thing I tell midwifery students is, individualise your approach. Start with the woman and what she feels the issue is." (Caroline, midwife)

Several people said they make a point of not mentioning someone's size or shape in any way, while others said that they actively looked for opportunities to point out positives and to use empowering language, for example about how babies looked so comfortable.

Many midwives stress the importance of trusting women's instincts, and of considering ergonomics.

"It's ergonomics. If I was supporting a woman who had one arm, or who had visual difficulties, or any person who doesn't fit in with the textbook picture example of breastfeeding (which is most women!), I would still ask the same questions to enable me to help support her feeding experience, because the fundamentals are the same: What positions feel good? What is comfortable for her and the baby? What is working for her and the baby? How does she feel about it?" (Katie James)

"It's about focusing on them as an individual and seeing what they need. If they need the baby in a different position, well fine, let's work that out. Plenty of women who are so-called average need that, for other reasons. We need to stop fat shaming women, even by accident, and focus on the human need to have good, kind, caring support to help you learn to breastfeed." (Millie, midwife)

Again, holistic assessment is important here, and this isn't just important for those with a higher BMI, but for anyone who needs help with breastfeeding.

"Does she have a long body or a short torso? Does she have a sore perineum, so she cannot sit upright for long in a chair at present? Where do her nipples point? It's not all about a woman's size when assisting with breastfeeding, it's about individualising care to that mother baby dyad. You could have a woman who's a size eight and she has smaller breasts with one nipple that points upwards and one out sideways, for example; we'd need to find the best ergonomic positions for breastfeeding for her too. With every mother baby dyad we should be assessing what might work for them and using all our senses to support that." (Katie James)

When supporting someone to breastfeed, it is important to consider time, sleep and the energy levels of both the mother and baby. Some women have long labours, and babies can sometimes be sleepy as the result of pain relief used during labour and birth. Trying to persuade a sleepy baby to feed can be counterproductive and lead to people feeling discouraged.

Weigh up the individual situation and the priorities, and consider when the optimal time for feeding support might be.

Explain the problems with the idea that there is some kind of 'normal', that we all have the same size breasts, that we can all feed in the same position, or that what we see in images of breastfeeding is some kind of ideal, because it actually only depicts a very narrow range of possibilities.

Breastfeeding, weight and the bigger picture

Although we have long been told that breastfeeding helps us lose weight after birth, I mentioned earlier that this isn't straightforward either, and I want to come back to this because it leads into a really important wider point.

The modern, western medical approach is based on old, outdated views of weight loss. It doesn't take into account other issues, such as stress, inequality, mental and physical health, and things like whether women are getting enough vitamins and minerals. Amy Brown explains why the idea that breastfeeding is directly correlated with weight loss is incorrect, which brings us back to some of the issues at the very root of the way our culture has misunderstood some of the fundamentals around weight and size.

"We know that producing breastmilk has a calorific need of around 500 calories a day. So, although we know that it's not as straightforward as the myth of 'calories in, calories out' suggests, some women may find that their body loses weight. This will be the women who have lower stress, aren't depressed, and aren't being fat shamed. Their hormones are working well, and they're responding well to the hormones of breastfeeding but they're not dieting, which is the key bit.

"But the body is designed to want to hold onto weight. From an evolutionary perspective, it doesn't want you to lose loads of weight, because that's savings in the bank. And I think that's particularly true when you've just had a baby. Evolution wouldn't want us to lose weight, so it's going to hang onto that as much as possible. So what I've learnt recently is that, if you expend too many calories

compared to what you're eating, then your body wonders what's going on, it will slow your metabolism down and stop doing things like repairs to your body. When I wasn't eating enough for the amount of exercise I was doing, I was wondering why I was losing my hair, and scars weren't healing. Your body stops all of that.

"So if you have a woman who has been told that she needs to lose weight and she starts dieting, her body is going to prioritise making breastmilk, but she's going to feel really crap and probably won't lose weight because her body is panicking, going 'I need to preserve all of this, she's not eating enough and we've got to feed that baby.' So she's told that it will help her lose weight but she doesn't lose any because her body's in panic mode. But for the woman who's got a BMI of 22 and everyone's like, 'oh, you've just snapped back to a healthy weight, let's say you're wonderful', and who is not dieting and who's eating enough for her baby, she'll probably start losing a bit of weight because she's not dieting. So breastfeeding does use calories, it's just that your body is very, very clever at adapting to that. And all those messages are just diet culture.

"The message that breastfeeding will help you lose weight is still there. But why on earth are we talking about that in antenatal classes? It might help you reduce some of the fat stores that you put on in pregnancy, because your body put them there because it was expecting to breastfeed, but only as long as you carry on eating in a healthy, nutritious way and meet your own calorie needs. If you start restricting food, your body will react." (Amy Brown)

The conversation that Amy and I had around how the body deprioritises activities like scar healing also led me to wonder about the statistic I shared earlier in this chapter which shows that larger women are more likely to have wound infections and take longer to heal. This is a very real, concrete example of where the reason for this may not be wholly about being larger. It may be partly or entirely the result of society's approach to larger people. Some larger women are either dieting or recovering from the effects of dieting. We know that dieting leads our bodies to divert energy from what it considers less essential processes, such as wound healing. These primal parts of our bodies don't know about caesareans; they're just trying to keep us safe, in the only ways they know how. But the net result is that our health suffers. Worse, the suffering is blamed on our size and alleged laziness, not on the fact that the relationships between weight, size, shape, and health have long been fundamentally misunderstood.

This is yet another example of where the western medical view of disease doesn't serve us well. I have said it before, but we need to take a different perspective; one that is informed by what we have learned over the past few decades about our bodies, our health, and the culture and structures that affect them. It is clear that we still have a lot to learn.

Tips for optimising your postnatal experience

The tips in this section offer a brief summary of some of the things that you can do to optimise your health after having a baby and reduce your chance of problems.

Whether or not you decide to have blood thinning medication, be aware of the symptoms of a blood clot (VTE). These include throbbing or cramping pain, swelling, warm, red, darkened, or painful skin around the affected area, and swollen veins which hurt when you touch them. Blood clots usually occur in the calf or thigh, but they can also develop in other places, such as the arm or tummy. With a blood clot, the pain, swelling and redness will almost always just be in one leg (or arm), rather than both. Always seek advice from a midwife, nurse or doctor straight away. If you have chest pain or are breathless, call the emergency services immediately, as these are symptoms of a blood clot having moved to your lungs (pulmonary embolism).

Just as we are advised to move around when we fly, mobilising can help reduce the chance of blood clots. This is especially the case if you've had a caesarean, but it's important for everyone. Change position frequently, try to move at least once an hour, and be especially mindful of not keeping your legs in the same position for too long.

Hydrate, hydrate, hydrate! It's so important to get lots of

fluid, both for your general wellbeing, and because this helps to prevent blood clots developing. Get yourself one of those water bottles with a built-in straw, so that you can drink in (almost) any position, and an insulated travel mug if you like hot drinks. Your tea is then less likely to go cold as you attend to the needs of your baby and any older children. If you're trying to find a gift for a new mum, these are perfect.

Even if you don't feel able to do much, it can be helpful to the body and the spirit to get some fresh air at least once a day. That doesn't mean you have to go and see anyone or do anything. If it's all you can manage, have a cup of tea in your garden, walk around the house, or get someone to help you into a car and take you for a drive.

If you have a wound, either from a caesarean or from stitches in your perineum, follow the tips in the wound healing section and expose it to air several times a day. I will again acknowledge that this is inelegant, no matter your shape or size, but it can help, and nobody else needs to see.

Wear clothes that aren't going to make you hotter, and in fact wear as little as you need to for those first few days. That means you're getting skin to skin with your baby as well. It doesn't matter what anybody else thinks. Just tell them you're not able to receive visitors yet. These are critical days for you, your baby and your family, so prioritise what you need.

Get support from appropriately qualified people. This might include help with housework, cleaning or child care, professional breastfeeding support, or health or wellness care for yourself. It may seem like an indulgence, especially if you are on a low income but, if you can afford it, it's well worth it. If you want to breastfeed, the initial cost of a lactation consultant, for instance, can lead to significant savings later, because this can help you avoid spending significant amounts of money on bottles and formula milk. There are often services available for those on a low income if you do some research or ask around.

Your health and wellbeing are important, and need to be prioritised, so that you can care for your baby well.

8. Conclusion

It seems quite clear from the evidence that BMI is a crude and outdated tool which is not useful as a means of predicting health by determining risk status. Having a higher BMI in itself doesn't equate to a high risk pregnancy, and focusing on BMI as a risk factor is an unhelpful, unevidenced and harmful approach to caring for pregnant women. It's true that having a high BMI is associated with an increased chance of experiencing some things, and a lower chance of experiencing others, both in pregnancy and more widely. However, association is only ever about population-level data. Many plus size women will not personally experience any of the things that I have discussed in this book. And yet, if they receive care within the maternity services, they will be subject to ongoing risk assessment, weight stigma, additional tests, interventions and restrictions simply because of their size.

Where poorer health outcomes are sometimes experienced in pregnancy and in general by those with a higher BMI, the evidence does not prove that this is linked to the physical effects of carrying additional weight. It is likely that these outcomes result at least partly from fatphobia and weight-based discrimination and the poorer quality of medical care that plus size people experience. Sadly, our ability to understand some aspects of this area more deeply has long been limited by the approach that western medicine has taken in this area.

"Until all research can control for weight cycling and weight stigma, we can't say that being at the higher end of the BMI spectrum causes any health conditions – even if higher weights are associated with these conditions." (Harrison 2019: 146)

My examination of the evidence on higher BMI and birth has also shown how the individual tests, restrictions and interventions suggested for plus size women may not be beneficial to women, babies and families. In some situations, there is evidence that we are doing more harm than good.

It is beyond time that we realised that BMI is not the measurement that matters the most; that we need to take a wider, more holistic approach to the care of plus size women.

When it comes to pregnancy, some important questions need to be asked. If a woman with a higher BMI hasn't developed pre-eclampsia or gestational diabetes in pregnancy, then why is she being treated as 'high risk'? Why are we not spending as much time telling plus size women about the advantages that their BMI brings? These include less chance of having a preterm birth, a lower risk of experiencing a compromising postpartum haemorrhage, less chance of having a serious tear, and potentially having more reserves to cope if you have a longer labour. And why, when there is so much evidence that midwifery-led care which focuses on physiology and takes a more respectful approach can significantly improve outcomes for women with a higher BMI, are those things not being prioritised?

So what can you do?

So what can you do now that you know what the evidence really says about higher BMI and birth? Some people may be able to use this information to improve their quality of care. I don't want to suggest that this is always possible for everybody, in every situation, because to do so would be to ignore the effect of the very inequalities that I have been discussing throughout this book. But for some of the people who live in a larger body, there are some things you can do to make your life and pregnancy journey easier.

For instance, now that you are aware of the negative effects of weight-based discrimination, and that social media is a major cause of negative body image (Hicks & Brown 2016), you may wish to do some more reading, and curate your social media feeds while also seeking out positive ways of learning more about other approaches. I have mentioned several books which I would highly recommend.

There are also some decisions you can proactively make to

help navigate your way through pregnancy and birth within a medical system. You may also want to explore and consider options such as giving birth outside of the system, at home, or in another midwifery-led setting. You can use the information in this book as a basis for conversations with care providers. The book itself can be a way of opening conversations about your care and the information you are being given: ask your midwife, doctor, doula, and childbirth educator if they have read it.

I hope I have shown that one key to having the kind of birth you want is to do everything in your power to get the right people around you, and to plan to give birth in an environment which will support you and your physiology. This is important for everyone, but it can be particularly important for those with a higher BMI. It is abundantly clear from the evidence that healthy plus size women have a far higher chance of a straightforward pregnancy and birth and a good outcome if they stay away from very medical settings and opt for a more low-tech, personalised alternative.

In maternity care, standardisation, or the application of the same frameworks, pathways and care packages across the board, is deemed the best approach. But this leads to the creation of universal rules and rigid guidelines that leave little room for thinking or individualised care. We can see how this isn't working in the care of plus size women. So get informed, get support, and get educated. Consider how to find people and ways to help you forge your own path, build your confidence, and trust your instincts and decisions. Be open to considering alternatives, even if they would not have been your first choice before.

I noticed a fascinating parallel while I was writing this book. I mentioned in chapter seven that one of the most promising approaches to tackling the negative effects of diet culture is something called 'intuitive eating'. This is an approach which helps people re-learn to trust their bodies. It's vital that we explore ideas like this, because those profiting from diet culture have benefitted from teaching us that we cannot trust ourselves, and that we instead should buy their latest diet book, course, food, pill, supplement, surgery, weight loss or wellness programme, or – hot off the press – fabulous new weight loss injection. It struck me recently that I have spent nearly three decades writing about how the problems that we see in maternity care also stem from the very same profit-driven approach, which also works by encouraging reliance on monitoring, tests, interventions, tools, courses, and other external 'solutions' rather than on listening to one's own body and instincts. These are both examples of capitalism at its finest, in the sense that we are being taught from a very early age that we are inadequate and therefore need to spend our money on solutions that will improve or fix us, while making others rich.

Why we all need to keep exploring...

Despite a lack of evidence that being larger is a genuine problem in and of itself, the idea that BMI is a problem remains deeply embedded in maternity care. Groups of self-appointed experts have encoded their opinions into written form in documents which have become guidance that dictates the experience of millions of women. It's unconscionable that we have to defend ourselves against a medical system that purports to help us. But this isn't just a problem in maternity care. It's a much wider problem.

We have an incredibly long way to go in further exploring and undoing the negative effects of weight bias and our cultural approach to people with a higher BMI. As Harrison (2019: 49) concludes, *"diet culture is a system of oppression with racist, sexist roots,"* and we all have a part to play in dismantling this. I've been reminded as I was writing this book that some of the most otherwise enlightened people exhibit weight bias and fatphobia. For instance, some of the researchers who I know from my exploration of topics like induction of labour to be very woman-centred are far less likely to question assumptions and beliefs when it comes to research relating to weight and pregnancy. This is also noted by Flint and Reale (2014), who wrote to *The Lancet* about their experience of hearing fatphobic, stereotyping, and insulting remarks from renowned presenters at a large conference for the study of obesity in the UK.

This prejudice is also clear in written research papers. The suggested interventions are not questioned as strongly, the language is often judgemental, and the assumptions that underlie weight bias are not challenged in the same way as those which relate to interventions such as induction of labour, intrapartum antibiotics, or early cord clamping. This suggests that, on some level, the researchers have weight bias and believe in some of the harmful, unevidenced ideas about size and health that scientists now know to be false.

That's not surprising. The diet industry relies on people not thinking too deeply about these issues. So I know that some of the people who read this book will be encountering the concept of 'diet culture' for the first time. You may not have previously realised that the people around you, perhaps including some of those you love, are transmitting messages that may be causing you harm. Perhaps you've been believing some of them yourself.

It might be that you picked this book up simply to find out whether you truly needed to have heparin injections, or how you could get to use a birth pool despite having a higher BMI, and didn't expect to be hit with the bigger picture that I've discussed. If that's the case and you are now realising that you have been negatively affected by the myths and stigma that surround ideas about weight, then I offer a virtual hug alongside some gentle encouragement to keep reading. Don't let this be the end of your exploration.

My reason for making this request is that I'm really aware that I have merely scratched the surface of this topic in order to put what I wanted to say about maternity care into a context. There are many amazing books, people, social media accounts, and organisations out there from which you can learn more. Knowledge truly is power, and I want to encourage you to continue to read, learn, and connect with others working in this area, for this can help you to unravel the unhealthy messages that we've all been subject to and which have been so harmful to so many of us.

If you're not sure where to start, then some of the key phrases to start looking for are Health at Every Size (HAES) and intuitive eating. If you want to know more about the problem first, try searching on diet culture, and have a look at some of the books in the reference list. Some of the most valuable ones (in my opinion) to read next if you're new to this area and want more detail and evidence are those by Bacon (2008), Harrison (2019) and Wolrich (2021). To learn more about how diet culture affects Black and Brown women, look up Strings (2015, 2019). For an unapologetically loud and sweary take on loving your larger body, see Baker's (2015) *Things no-one will tell fat girls* and Hagen's (2020) *Happy Fat*. For birth stories and a positive, joyful approach to pregnancy in a larger body, see Mayefske (2021). Many of these authors have websites and are on social media as well, although the sad reality is that people get so much abuse for speaking out on this topic that they often need to close accounts and make new ones, so it's better for you to search than for me to offer links that might be out of date by the time you read this.

I want to urge readers who aren't living in larger bodies to keep reading and researching as well, for so many reasons. Even if you value physical attractiveness and fit our current cultural physical idea of what that looks like, that might not always be the case. It's also the case that people you care about who do fit that ideal are being harmed by diet culture and its associated messages just as much as those who don't. I hope that you will also use the reference list in this book to seek out the positive books, people, accounts, and resources that can help you and those you love.

I also hope you will consider how you consume plus size pregnancy health 'advice' on the internet. This isn't because I don't want anyone to research. Quite the opposite. But, as I was writing this book, I discovered an astonishing amount of misinformation online. Probably more so than for any other topic that I have researched and, more worryingly, some of it is put out by organisations and people that I would usually trust. It seems as if even those people who question the routine use of other tests, restrictions, and interventions are happy to accept the tenets of diet culture, and the idea that being larger is a significant risk factor. As a result, there is less questioning of the recommendations and a lot more mindless repetition of some of the myths that I have unpacked in this book and shown to be false.

If you are a health care provider or birth worker, please use the reference list to further educate yourself and question whether the recommendations that underpin the care you give are evidence-based, reasonable, and compassionate.

If you consider yourself a holistic or 'alternative' birth worker, please don't think that you are immune from this. You're not. Birth workers may not be actively promoting weight management groups or glucose tolerance tests, and they may be up in arms about low molecular weight heparin or the restrictions that larger women face when they want to access birth pools within systems of maternity care, but many discuss or allude to topics such as body image, weight, diet, and nutrition without a deep understanding of how some of the messages that they are sharing perpetuate diet culture. I hear women talking about how some childbirth educators only ever depict slim women in their materials, which sends an unspoken message. And I would invite you to consider whether you make comments in the presence of women and families about your own eating or dieting habits, for instance remarking that you are 'naughty' for eating chocolate, or suggesting that you need to go on a diet because you ate too much on holiday. Such comments can also reinforce and perpetuate some of our cultural myths about size, weight, and related issues which, as you now know, aren't evidence-based and can be harmful.

Remember that body image and how somebody feels about themselves and their body is a stronger predictor of health than body size (Harrison 2019).

It's not just about larger bodies, though. It's about caring for and supporting *all* bodies. A few years ago, I was teaching a workshop with midwives and we got onto the topic of caring for plus size women. A few of the larger midwives in the room got into a joking conversation during part of the session and someone made a comment about 'skinny' midwives, which got a laugh. At which point a slim midwife gently pointed out that she was no more able to put on weight than some of her larger friends were able to lose it, and that it's just as unhelpful and inappropriate to make jokes about smaller, slimmer people. She was absolutely right. We need to co-create a world that is welcoming to people of ALL shapes and sizes. We need a culture in which we can develop a view of health that is truly individual and encompassing of the factors that are actually relevant and evidence-based, while moving away from an unevidenced focus on size and shape, particularly when this is often influenced by political and economic interests. We need compassion, for ourselves and for each other.

I'd like to sign off this book with an important reminder. The vast majority of women who have a higher BMI are more than capable of experiencing a healthy, happy pregnancy, a straightforward, physiological labour and birth, and a joyful (if sometimes tiring, but that's not about size!) start to life as a new parent. The majority of plus size women will not experience problems, especially if they opt for woman-centred caregivers and settings. You do not have to accept any label that doesn't suit your needs. You are strong, capable, and wonderful, no matter what your size, shape, or weight. You can be a fabulous parent, a healthy person, and somebody totally worthy of love, respect, and excellent health care at any size. Please don't believe anybody who tries to tell you otherwise. They clearly haven't read the evidence.

To see more of Sara's work:

Visit my website at www.sarawickham.com

Sign up for my free monthly newsletter and get information on new books, courses and projects at www.sarawickham.com/news

If you have enjoyed this book and found it useful, please leave a review at your favourite book retailer - it really helps highlight it to others who might need it.

Other books by Sara which you might enjoy:

In Your Own Time: how western medicine controls the start of labour and why this needs to stop
Inducing Labour: making informed decisions
Anti-D Explained
Group B Strep Explained
Vitamin K and the Newborn
What's Right for Me? Making decisions in pregnancy and childbirth
Birthing Your Placenta: the third stage of labour
101 tips for planning, writing and surviving your dissertation

References

Abalos E, Cuesta C, Grosso AL *et al* (2013). Global and regional estimates of preeclampsia and eclampsia. EJOGRB 170: 1-7.

ACOG (2018). ACOG Practice Bulletin no 196: Thromboembolism in Pregnancy. O&G 132(1): e1-e17.

ACOG (2021). ACOG Practice Bulletin no 230: Obesity in Pregnancy. O&G 137(6): 1137-39.

Al-Zirqi I, Daltveit AK, Forsen L *et al* (2017). Risk factors for complete uterine rupture. AJOG 216(2): 165 e1-e8.

Anon (2020). Ending weight bias and the stigma of obesity. Nat Rev Endocrinol 16(5): 253.

Antonopoulos AS & Tousoulis D (2017). The molecular mechanisms of obesity paradox. Cardiovasc Res 113(9): 1074-86.

Ashwell M & Gibson S (2016). Waist-to-height ratio as an indicator of 'early health risk': simpler and more predictive than using a 'matrix' based on BMI and waist circumference. BMJ Open 6(3): e010159.

Association of Life Insurance Medical Directors: Medico-actuarial mortality investigations. ALIMD and Actuarial Soc Am 1912:1.

Atkinson L, Shaw RL, French DP *et al* (2016). Is pregnancy a teachable moment for diet and physical activity behaviour change? An interpretative phenomenological analysis of the experiences of women during their first pregnancy. B J Hlth Psych 21(4): 842-58.

Atkinson L, French DP, Ménage D *et al* (2017). Midwives' experiences of referring obese women to either a community or home-based antenatal weight management service: Implications for service providers and midwifery practice. Midwifery 49: 102-09.

Aughey H, Jardine J, Moitt N *et al* (2021). Waterbirth: a national retrospective cohort study of factors associated with its use among women in England. BMC P&C 21: 256.

Australasian Diabetes in Pregnancy Society (ADIPS) (2014). ADIPS Consensus Guidelines for the Testing and Diagnosis of Hyperglycaemia in Pregnancy in Australia and New Zealand. bit.ly/3KyxfH9

Australian Bureau of Statistics (2019). National Aboriginal and Torres Strait Islander Health Survey. bit.ly/3MBEuRd

Australian Institute of Health and Welfare (2022a). Australia's Mothers and Babies. bit.ly/3GEMRre

Australian Institute of Health and Welfare (2022b). Maternal deaths. bit.ly/3Uu2lEp

Bacon L (2008). Health at Every Size. The surprising truth about your weight. Dallas: BenBella Books.

Bacon L & Aphromor L (2011). Weight Science: Evaluating the Evidence for a Paradigm Shift. Nutrition Journal 10(1): 9.

Baer RJ, Chambers BD, Coleman-Phox K *et al* (2022). Risk of early birth by body mass index in a propensity score-matched sample: A retrospective cohort study. BJOG 2022; 129: 1704-11.

Baker J (2015). Things no-one will tell fat girls. New York: Seal Press.

Barau G, Robillard PY, Hulsey TC *et al* (2006). Linear association between maternal pre-pregnancy body mass index and risk of cesarean section in term deliveries. BJOG 113(10): 1173-77.

Bartsch E, Medcalf KE, Park AL *et al* (2016). Clinical risk factors for pre-eclampsia determined in early pregnancy: systematic review and meta-analysis of large cohort studies. BMJ 353: i1753.

Beech B (2021). Am I Allowed? What every woman needs to know before she gives birth. Edinburgh: BPPF.

Begley CM, Gyte GML, Devane D *et al* (2019). Active versus expectant management for women in the third stage of labour. Cochrane Database Syst Rev 2019(2): CD007412.

Benfield RD, Hortobagyi T, Tanner CJ *et al* (2010). The effects of hydrotherapy on anxiety, pain, neuroendocrine responses, and contraction dynamics during labor. Biol Res Nurs 12(1): 28-36.

Beta J, Khan N, Khalil A *et al* (2019). Maternal and neonatal complications of fetal macrosomia: systematic review and meta-analysis. Ultrasound Obstet Gynecol 54(3): 308-18.

Betrán AP, Temmerman M, Kingdon C *et al* (2018). Interventions to reduce unnecessary caesarean sections in healthy women and babies. Lancet 392(10155): 1358-68.

Bhattacharya S, Campbell DM, Liston WA *et al* (2007). Effect of Body Mass Index on pregnancy outcomes in nulliparous women delivering singleton babies. BMC Public Health 7:168.

Bick D (2009). Addressing the obesity epidemic: Time for the maternity services to act now but what strategies should we use? Midwifery 25(4): 337-38.

Bick D, Taylor C, Bhavnani V *et al* (2020). Lifestyle information and commercial weight management groups to support maternal postnatal weight management and positive lifestyle behaviour: the SWAN feasibility randomised controlled trial. BJOG 127: 636-45.

Biesty LM, Egan AM, Dunne F *et al* (2018). Planned birth at or near term for improving health outcomes for pregnant women with gestational diabetes and their infants. Cochrane Database Syst Rev 2018(1): CD012910.

Blaylock R, Trickey H, Sanders J *et al* (2022). WRISK Voices: A mixed-methods study of women's experiences of pregnancy-related public health advice and risk messages in the UK. Midwifery 113: 103433.

Blomberg M (2011). Maternal obesity and risk of postpartum hemorrhage. O&G 118(3): 561-68.
Booker WA (2022). The effect of maternal obesity on labour. BJOG 129: 2175.
Boulvain M, Irion O, Dowswell T *et al* (2016). Induction of labour at or near term for suspected fetal macrosomia. Cochrane Database Syst Rev 2016(5): CD000938.
Brocato B, Lewis D, Mulekar M *et al* (2019). Obesity's impact on intrapartum electronic fetal monitoring. JM-FNM 32(1): 92-94.
Brown A (2019). Informed is Best. How to spot fake news about your pregnancy, birth and baby. London: Pinter and Martin.
Brown A (2021). Breastfeeding Uncovered. Second Edition. London: Pinter and Martin.
Brown A, Rance J & Warren L (2015). Body image concerns during pregnancy are associated with a shorter breast feeding duration. Midwifery 31(1): 80-89.
Brown PJ & Konner M (1987). An anthropological perspective on obesity. Ann NY Acad Sci 499: 29-46.
Brzecka A & Ejma M (2015). Obesity paradox in the course of cerebrovascular diseases. Adv Clin Exp Med 24(3): 379-83.
Buckley S (2015). Hormonal physiology of childbearing: evidence and implications for women, babies, & maternity care. JPerEd 24(3): 145-53.
Burns E, Feeley C, Hall PJ *et al* (2022). Systematic review and meta-analysis to examine intrapartum interventions, and maternal and neonatal outcomes following immersion in water during labour and waterbirth. BMJ Open 12:e056517.
Burton G J, Redman C W, Roberts J M *et al* (2019). Pre-eclampsia: pathophysiology and clinical implications. BMJ 366: l2381
Butwick AJ, Bentley J, Leonard SA *et al* (2019). Prepregnancy maternal body mass index and venous thromboembolism: a population-based cohort study. BJOG 126: 581-88.
Calix R, Silasi M, Lundsberg LS *et al* (2020). Maternal pre-pregnancy BMI and risk of preterm birth. AJOG 222(1): S577.
Carbone S, Lavie CJ & Arena R (2017). Obesity and heart failure: focus on the obesity paradox. Mayo Clin Proc 92(2): 266–79.
Carbone S, Canada JM, Billingsley HE *et al* (2019). Obesity paradox in cardiovascular disease. Vasc H Risk Man 15: 89-100.
Carlhäll S, Källén K & Blomberg M (2020). The effect of maternal body mass index on duration of induced labor. AOGS 99(5): 669-78.
Carlson NS, Corwin EJ & Lowe NK (2017). Labor intervention and outcomes in women who are nulliparous and obese: comparison of nurse-midwife to obstetrician intrapartum care. JMWH 62(1): 29-39.
Caro JF, Sinha MK, Kolaczynski JW *et al* (1996). Leptin: the tale of an obesity gene. Diabetes. 45(11): 1455-62.

Cedergren MI (2004). Maternal morbid obesity and the risk of adverse pregnancy outcome. O&G 103(2): 219-24.
Cedergren MI (2009). Non-elective caesarean delivery due to ineffective uterine contractility or due to obstructed labour in relation to maternal body mass index. EJOGRB 145: 163-66.
Champion ML, Jauk VC, Biggio JR *et al* (2022). Early Gestational Diabetes Screening Based on ACOG Guidelines. Am J Perinat doi: 10.1055/a-1925-1134.
Chauhan SP, Grobman WA, Gherman RA *et al* (2005). Suspicion and treatment of the macrosomic fetus. AJOG 193(2): 332-46.
Cheng ER, Declercq ER, Belanoff C *et al* (2015). Labor and delivery experiences of mothers with suspected large babies. MCHJ 19(12):2578-86.
Christenson A, Torgerson J & Hemmingsson E (2020). Attitudes and beliefs in Swedish midwives and obstetricians towards obesity and gestational weight management. BMC P&C 20(1):755.
Clark SL (2022). Category II Intrapartum fetal heart rate patterns unassociated with recognized sentinel events. Castles in the air. O&G 139(6): 1003-08.
Clark-Ganheart CA, Reddy UM, Kominiarek MA *et al* (2015). Pregnancy Outcomes Among Obese Women and Their Offspring by Attempted Mode of Delivery. O&G 126(5): 987-93.
Cluett ER, Burns E, Cuthbert A (2018). Immersion in water during labour and birth. Cochrane Database Syst Rev 2018(5): CD000111.
Cnossen JS, Leeflang MM, de Haan EE *et al* (2007). Accuracy of body mass index in predicting pre-eclampsia: bivariate meta-analysis. BJOG 114: 1477–85.
Coates D, Makris A, Catling C *et al* (2020). A systematic scoping review of clinical indications for induction of labour. Plos One 15(1): e0228196.
Coelho HF, Murray L, Royal-Lawson M *et al* (2011) Antenatal anxiety disorder as a predictor of postnatal depression: a longitudinal study. J Affect Dis 129(1): 348-53.
Colson S (2019). Biological Nurturing. London: Pinter and Martin.
Constable L, Monga D, Mylonas G *et al* (2020), The impact of maternal body mass index on the rate of obstetric anal sphincter injury in nulliparous women. ANZJOG 60: 514-21.
Cook TM, Woodall N & Frerk C (2011). Major complications of airway management in the UK: results of the Fourth National Audit Project of the Royal College of Anaesthetists and the Difficult Airway Society. Part 1: anaesthesia. Br J Anaesth 106(5): 617-31.
Coxon K, Homer C, Bisits A *et al* (2016) 'Reconceptualising risk in childbirth'. Midwifery 38: 1-5.
Crane SC, Wojtowycz MA, Dye TD *et al* (1997). Association between pre-pregnancy obesity and the risk of cesarean. O&G 89(2): 213-16.

Crawford D, Jeffery RW & French SA (2000). Can anyone successfully control their weight? Findings of a three year community-based study of men and women. Int J Obes Rel Met Dis 24(9):1107-10.

Creanga AA, Syverson C, Seed K *et al* (2017). Pregnancy-Related Mortality in the United States, 2011-2013. O&G 130(2): 366-73.

Crequit S, Korb D, Morin C *et al* (2020). Use of the Robson classification to understand the increased risk of cesarean section in case of maternal obesity. BMC P&C 20(1): 738.

Cryle P & Stephens E (2017). Normality: A Critical Genealogy. Chicago: University of Chicago Press.

Daemers D, Wijnen H, van Limbeek E *et al* (2014). The impact of obesity on outcomes of midwife-led pregnancy and childbirth in a primary care population. BJOG. 121: 1403–14.

Dahlen HG, Thornton C, Downe S *et al* (2021). Intrapartum interventions and outcomes for women and children following induction of labour at term in uncomplicated pregnancies: a 16-year population-based linked data study. BMJ Open 11:e047040

Dalbye R, Gunnes N, Blix E *et al* (2021). Maternal body mass index and risk of obstetric, maternal and neonatal outcomes: A cohort study of nulliparous women with spontaneous onset of labor. AOGS 100(3): 521-30.

Das S & Ungoed-Thomas J (2023). Maker of Wegovy 'skinny jab' is funding NHS weight-loss services. Guardian bit.ly/415sUC7

Davey MA & King J (2016). Caesarean section following induction of labour in uncomplicated first births- a population-based cross-sectional analysis of 42,950 births. BMC P&C 16: 92.

Dawe JP, McCowan LME, Wilson J *et al* (2020). Probiotics and Maternal Mental Health: A Randomised Controlled Trial among Pregnant Women with Obesity. Sci Rep 10(1): 1291.

Declerq E, MacDorman M, Osterman M *et al* (2015). Prepregnancy obesity and primary cesareans among otherwise low-risk mothers in 38 U.S. states in 2012. Birth 42: 4.

DeJoy SB & Bittner K (2015). Obesity Stigma as a Determinant of Poor Birth Outcomes in Women with High BMI: A Conceptual Framework. MCHJ 19(4): 693-99.

Denison FC, Aedla NR, Keag O *et al* (2018). Care of women with obesity in pregnancy. Green-top guideline 72. BJOG. 126(3):e62-e106.

Denison F, Price J, Graham C *et al* (2008). Maternal obesity, length of gestation, risk of postdates pregnancy and spontaneous onset of labour at term. BJOG 115: 720-25.

De-Regil L, Peña-Rosas J, Fernández-Gaxiola AC *et al* (2015). Effects and safety of periconceptional oral folate supplementation for preventing birth defects. Cochrane Database Syst Rev 2015(12): CD007950.

Ding X, Wu Y, Xu S *et al* (2014) Maternal anxiety during pregnancy and adverse birth outcomes: a systematic review and meta-analysis of prospective cohort studies. J Affect Dis 159: 103-10.

Dodd JM, Grivell RM, Deussen AR *et al* (2018). Metformin for women who are overweight or obese during pregnancy for improving maternal and infant outcomes. Cochrane Database Syst Rev 2018(7): CD010564.

Donnelly L & Taylor R (2023). Midwives should end 'terrible' links with Slimming World over concerns for mothers' mental health. bit.ly/3MIbfvZ

Driessen M, Bouvier-Colle M-H, Dupont C *et al* (2011). Postpartum hemorrhage resulting from uterine atony after vaginal delivery: factors associated with severity. O&G 117(1): 21–31.

D'Souza R, Horyn I, Jacob CE *et al* (2021). Birth outcomes in women with body mass index of 40 kg/m² or greater stratified by planned and actual mode of birth. AOGS 100(2): 200-09.

Duley L, Meher S, Hunter KE *et al* (2019). Antiplatelet agents for preventing pre-eclampsia and its complications. Cochrane Database Syst Rev 2019(10): CD004659.

Dunkel Schetter C, Niles AN, Guardino CM *et al* (2016). Demographic, Medical, and Psychosocial Predictors of Pregnancy Anxiety. Paed Perinat Epid 30(5): 421-29.

Durnwald CP, Ehrenberg HM & Mercer BM (2004). The impact of maternal obesity and weight gain on vaginal birth after cesarean section success. AJOG 191: 954-57.

Dwyer ER, Filion KB, MacFarlane AJ *et al* (2022). Who should consume high-dose folic acid supplements before and during early pregnancy for the prevention of neural tube defects? BMJ 377: e067728.

Edwards N (2019). Birthing Your Baby: the second stage of labour. Edinburgh: BPPF.

Edwards N & Wickham S (2018). Birthing Your Placenta: the third stage of labour. Avebury: Birthmoon Creations.

Elagizi A, Kachur S, Lavie CJ *et al* (2018). An Overview and Update on Obesity and the Obesity Paradox in Cardiovascular Diseases. Prog Cardiovasc Dis. 61(2): 142-150.

Ellekjaer KL, Bergholt T & Løkkegaard E (2017). Maternal obesity and its effect on labour duration in nulliparous women: a retrospective observational cohort study. BMC P&C 17:222.

Ellis JA, Brown CM, Barger B *et al* (2019). Influence of Maternal Obesity on Labor Induction: A Systematic Review and Meta-Analysis. JMWH 64(1): 55-67.

Ellison J, McPhail D & Mitchinson W (Eds) (2016). Obesity in Canada: Critical Perspectives. University of Toronto Press.

Eloranta A-M, Gunnarsdottir I, Thorisdottir B *et al* (2023) The combined effect of pre-pregnancy body mass index and gestational weight gain on the risk of pre-labour and intrapartum caesarean section – The ICE-MCH study. PLoS ONE 18(1): e0280060.
Evans B & Colls R (2009). Measuring fatness, governing bodies: The spatialities of the body mass index (BMI) in anti-obesity politics. Antipode 41(5): 1051–83.
Farrar D, Duley L, Dowswell T *et al* (2017). Different strategies for diagnosing gestational diabetes to improve maternal and infant health. Cochrane Database Syst Rev 2017(8): CD007122.
Ferres MA, Olivarez SA, Trinh V *et al* (2011). Rate of wound complications with enoxaparin use among women at high risk for postpartum thrombosis. O&G 117: 119–24.
Fildes A, Charlton J, Rudisill C *et al* (2015). Probability of an obese person attaining normal body weight: Cohort study using electronic health records. Am J Pub Hlth 105(9): e54-9.
Fitzpatrick KE, Kurinczuk JJ, Alfirevic Z *et al* (2012). Uterine rupture by intended mode of delivery in the UK: a national case-control study. PLoS Med. 9(3): e1001184.
Flegal K, Graubard B, Williamson D *et al* (2005) Excess deaths associated with underweight, overweight, and obesity. JAMA 293(15): 1861–67.
Flessa HC, Kapstrom AB, Glueck HI *et al* (1965). Placental transport of heparin. AJOG 93: 570–73.
Flint SW & Reale S (2014). Obesity stigmatisation from obesity researchers. The Lancet 384(9958): 1925-26.
Furber CM & McGowan L (2011). A qualitative study of the experiences of women who are obese and pregnant in the UK. Midwifery 27(4): 437-44.
Fyfe EM, Thompson JM, Anderson NH *et al* (2012). Maternal obesity and postpartum haemorrhage after vaginal and caesarean delivery among nulliparous women at term. BMC P&C 12: 112.
Gallagher D, Visser M, Sepulveda D *et al* (1996). How Useful Is Body Mass Index for Comparison of Body Fatness across Age, Sex, and Ethnic Groups? Am J Epid 143: 228-39.
Ganz ML, Wintfeld N, Li Q *et al* (2014). The association of body mass index with the risk of type 2 diabetes: a case–control study nested in an electronic health records system in the US. Diab Met Syn 6, 50.
Gard M (2008). Friends, enemies and the cultural politics of critical obesity research. In: Wright J and Harwood V (eds) Governing Bodies. London: Taylor and Francis, 31–44.
Gard M & Wright J (2005). The Obesity Epidemic: Science, Morality and Ideology. London: Routledge.

Gaudet L, Ferraro ZM, Wen SW *et al* (2014). Maternal obesity and occurrence of fetal macrosomia: a systematic review and meta-analysis. Biomed Res Int. 2014: 640291.

Glazer KB, Danilack VA, Field AE *et al* (2020). Term labor induction and cesarean delivery risk among obese women with and without comorbidities. A J Perinat doi: 10.1055/s-0040-1714422.

Goer H (2022). Do Epidurals Increase Cesareans? bit.ly/3JttUJK

Goer H & Romano A (2012). Optimal Care in Childbirth: The Case for a Physiologic Approach. Seattle, WA: Classic Day Publishing.

Goldenberg RL, Culhane JF, Iams JD *et al* (2008). Epidemiology and causes of preterm birth. Lancet 371(9606): 75-84.

Goldstein RF, Abell SK, Ranasinha S *et al* (2017). Association of gestational weight gain with maternal and infant outcomes: a systematic review and meta-analysis. JAMA 317(21): 2207-25.

Gray N, Picone G, Sloan F *et al* (2015). Relation between BMI and diabetes mellitus and its complications among US older adults. South Med J 108(1): 29-36.

Gross TL, Sokol RJ, Williams T *et al* (1987). Shoulder dystocia: a fetal-physician risk. AJOG 156: 1408–18.

Guh DP, Zhang W, Bansback N *et al* (2009). The incidence of co-morbidities related to obesity and overweight: a systematic review and meta-analysis. BMC Pub Health 9:88.

Guo Z, Liu L, Yu F *et al* (2021). The causal association between body mass index and type 2 diabetes mellitus-evidence based on regression discontinuity design. Diab Metab Res Rev 37(8): e3455.

Gupta S, Jeeyaselan S, Guleria R *et al* (2014). An observational study of various predictors of success of vaginal delivery following a previous cesarean section. JOG India 64(4): 260-64.

Gurol-Urganci I, Cromwell DA, Edozien LC *et al* (2013). Third- and fourth-degree perineal tears among primiparous women in England between 2000 and 2012. BJOG 120(12): 1516-25.

Haavaldsen C, Morken N-H, Saugstad OD *et al* (2023). Is the increasing prevalence of labor induction accompanied by changes in pregnancy outcomes? AOGS 102(2): 158-73.

Hagen S (2020). Happy Fat: Taking up space in a world that wants to shrink you. London: Fourth Estate.

Haines HM, Rubertson C, Pallant JF *et al* (2012) 'The influence of women's fear, attitudes and beliefs of childbirth on mode and experience of birth', BMC P&C 12(55): 1-14.

Hamm RF, Combs A & Davidson C (2020). SMFM Patient Safety Guideline: Reducing the risk of transmitting infection by transvaginal ultrasound examination. AJOG 223(3): PB3-B6.

Hamm RF, Teefey CP, Dolin CD *et al* (2021). Risk of cesarean delivery for women with obesity using a standardized labor induction protocol. A J Perinat DOI: 10.1055/s-0041-1732459
Harenberg J, Schneider D, Heilmann L *et al* (1993). Lack of anti-factor Xa activity in umbilical cord vein samples after subcutaneous administration of heparin or low molecular mass heparin in pregnant women. Haemostasis 23: 314–20.
Harrison C (2019). Anti-Diet. Reclaim your time, money, well-being and happiness through intuitive eating. London: Yellow Kite.
Harrison CL, Teede H, Khan N *et al* (2021). Weight management across preconception, pregnancy, and postpartum: A systematic review and quality appraisal of international clinical practice guidelines. Obesity Reviews 22(10): e13310.
Harvey L, vanElburg R & van der Beek EM (2021). Macrosomia and large for gestational age in Asia: one size does not fit all. JOGR 47: 1929-45.
Hautakangas T, Uotila J, Kontiainen J *et al* (2022). Impact of obesity on uterine contractile activity during labour: A blinded analysis of a randomised controlled trial cohort. BJOG 129: 1790-97.
Hegerty CK (2020). The new gestational diabetes: Treatment, evidence and consent. ANZJOG 60(3): 482-85.
Henderson J, Burns EE, Regalia AL *et al* (2014). Labouring women who used a birthing pool in obstetric units in Italy: prospective observational study. BMC P&C 14:17.
Hendler I, Goldenberg RL, Mercer BM *et al* (2005). The Preterm Prediction Study: association between maternal body mass index and spontaneous and indicated preterm birth. AJOG 192(3): 882-86.
Heslehurst N, Evans EH, Incollingo Rodriguez AC *et al* (2022). Newspaper media framing of obesity during pregnancy in the UK: A review and framework synthesis. Obes Rev 23(12): e13511.
Heslehurst N, Simpson H, Ells LJ *et al* (2008). The impact of maternal BMI status on pregnancy outcomes with immediate short-term obstetric resource implications: a meta-analysis. Obes Rev 9: 635–83.
Hibbard JU, Gilbert S, Landon MB *et al* (2006). Trial of labor or repeat cesarean delivery in women with morbid obesity and previous cesarean delivery. O&G 108: 125-33.
Hicks S & Brown A (2016). Higher Facebook use predicts greater body image dissatisfaction during pregnancy: The role of self-comparison. Midwifery 40: 132-140.
Hill IF, Angrish K, Nutter S *et al* (2023). Exploring body dissatisfaction in pregnancy and the association with gestational weight gain, obesity, and weight stigma. Midwifery 119: 103627.
Hoch M, Meloncelli N & de Jersey S (2023). Examining enhanced implementation of routine antenatal care practices to support healthy pregnancy weight gain. JMWH doi.org/10.1111/jmwh.13477

Hollowell J, Pillas D, Rowe R *et al* (2014). The impact of maternal obesity on intrapartum outcomes in otherwise low risk women: secondary analysis of the Birthplace national prospective cohort study. BJOG 121:343–55.

Huang HY, Chen HL & Feng LP (2017). Maternal obesity and the risk of neural tube defects in offspring. Obes Res Clin Pract 11(2): 188-97.

Hunt S & Symonds A (1995). The Social Meaning of Midwifery. Palgrave.

Hurst DJ, Schmuhl NB, Voils CI *et al* (2021). Prenatal care experiences among pregnant women with obesity in Wisconsin, United States: a qualitative quality improvement assessment. BMC P&C 21(1): 139.

Hutton EK, Reitsma A, Simioni J *et al* (2019). Perinatal or neonatal mortality among women who intend at the onset of labour to give birth at home compared to women of low obstetrical risk who intend to give birth in hospital: A systematic review and meta-analyses. E Clinical Medicine. 25(14): 59-70.

Incollingo Rodriguez AC, Smieszek SM, Nippert KE *et al* (2020). Pregnant and postpartum women's experiences of weight stigma in healthcare. BMC P&C 20(1): 499.

Izquierdo AG, Crujeiras AB, Casanueva FF *et al* (2019). Leptin, obesity, and leptin resistance: where are we 25 years later? Nut 11(11): 2704.

Jabak S & Hameed A (2020). Continuous intrapartum fetal monitoring in gestational diabetes, where is the evidence? JM-FNM 35(22): 4354-57.

Jevitt CM, Stapleton S, Deng Y *et al* (2021). Birth outcomes of women with obesity enrolled for care at freestanding birth centers in the United States. JMWH 66(1): 14-23.

Jones C & Jomeen J (2017). Women with a BMI ≥ 30kg/m² and their experience of maternity care: A meta ethnographic synthesis. Midwifery 53: 87-95.

Juhasz G, Gyamfi C, Gyamfi P *et al* (2005). Effect of body mass index and excessive weight gain on success of vaginal birth after cesarean delivery. O&G 106: 741-46.

Justin TA & Jette S (2022). "That chart ain't for us": How Black women understand 'obesity', health, and physical activity. Hlth 26(5): 605-21.

Juul LA, Hartwig TS, Ambye L *et al* (2020). Noninvasive prenatal testing and maternal obesity: A review. OGS 99(6): 744-50.

Källén B, Finnström O, Nygren K-G *et al* (2013). Maternal and fetal factors which affect fetometry: use of in vitro fertilization and birth register data. EJOGRB 170: 372–76.

Kang J, Baek S-E, Kim T *et al* (2012). Impact of Fat Obesity on Laparoscopic Total Mesorectal Excision: More Reliable Indicator than Body Mass Index. Int. J Colorectal Dis 27: 497–505.

Kashanian M, Sharifzadeh F & Jouhari S (2019). Relationship between pre pregnancy maternal body mass index (BMI) with birth weight, and spontaneous preterm delivery. EJOGRB 234: e19.

Kawakita T, Iqbal SN, Huang C-C *et al* (2017). Nonmedically indicated induction in morbidly obese women is not associated with an increased risk of cesarean delivery. AJOG 217(4):451.e1–e8.
Kerrigan A, Kingdon C, Cheyne H *et al* (2015). Obesity and normal birth: a qualitative study of clinician's management of obese pregnant women during labour. BMC P&C 15: 256.
Keys A, Aravanis C, Blackburn HW *et al* (1967). Epidemiological studies related to coronary heart disease: characteristics of men aged 40–59 in seven countries. Acta Med Scand Suppl 460: 360–64.
Keys A, Fidanza F, Karvonen M *et al* (1972) Indices of Relative Weight and Obesity. J Chronic Dis 25: 329-43.
Keys A, Fidanza F, Karvonen MJ *et al* (2014). Indices of Relative Weight and Obesity. Int J Epid 43(3): 655–65.
Kirkham M (1999). The culture of midwifery in the National Health Service in England. JAN 30: 732-39.
Kite J, Huang BH, Laird Y *et al* (2022). Influence and effects of weight stigmatisation in media: A systematic review. E Clin Med 48: 101464.
Knight M, Kenyon S, Brocklehurst P *et al* (2014). Saving Lives, Improving Mothers' Care - Lessons learned to inform future maternity care from the UK and Ireland. Confidential Enquiries 2009-2012. Oxford: NPEU.
Knight M, Bunch K, Patel R *et al* (2022). Saving Lives, Improving Mothers' Care. Lessons learned to inform maternity care from the UK and Ireland. Confidential Enquiries 2018-20. Oxford: NPEU.
Knight-Agarwal CR, Williams LT, Davis D *et al* (2016). The perspectives of obese women receiving antenatal care: A qualitative study of women's experiences. Women and Birth 29(2): 189-95.
Kojima M & Kangawa K (2005). Ghrelin: Structure and Function. Physiological Reviews 85(2): 495-522
Kominiarek MA, Cassimatis I, Peace J *et al* (2022). Peripartum care of persons with obesity: a scoping review of recommendations and practical tools for implementation. BMJ Open 12: e061430.
Kominiarek MA & Chauhan SP (2016). Obesity before, during, and after pregnancy: A review and comparison of five national guidelines. Am J Perinat 33(5): 433-41.
Kominiarek MA, VanVeldhuisen P, Hibbard J *et al* (2010). The maternal body mass index: a strong association with delivery route. AJOG 203: 264.e1-e7.
Kominiarek MA, Zhang J, VanVeldhuisen P *et al* (2011). Contemporary labor patterns: the impact of maternal BMI. AJOG 205: 244.e1–e8.
Kotaska A (2018). Postpartum venous thromboembolism prophylaxis may cause more harm than benefit: a critical analysis of international guidelines through an evidence-based lens. BJOG 125: 1109- 16.
Kotaska A (2021). Postpartum Heparin Thromboprophylaxis: More Harm Than Good. O&G 138(4): 527-29.

Krogh LQ, Boie S, Henriksen TB *et al* (2021). Induction of labour at 39 weeks versus expectant management in low-risk obese women: study protocol for a randomised controlled study. BMJ Open 12: e057688.

Kuehn BM (2020). Put an End to Obesity Stigma, International Panel Urges. JAMA. 323(15): 1435.

Kuhn TS (1962). The Structure of Scientific Revolutions. University of Chicago Press.

Kullinger M, Haglund B, Kieler H *et al* (2016). Effects of ultrasound pregnancy dating on neonatal morbidity in late preterm and early term male infants. BMC P&C 16(1): 1-8.

Kumari AS (2001). Pregnancy outcome in women with morbid obesity IJGO 73: 101-07.

Kurz CF & König AN (2020). The causal influence of maternal obesity on preterm birth. Lancet Diabetes Endocrinol 8(2): 101-03.

Lanier, AL, Wiegand SL, Fennig K *et al* (2021). Neonatal Outcomes After Delivery in Water. O&G 138(4): 622-26.

Leahy K, Berlin KS, Banks GG *et al* (2017). The relationship between intuitive eating and postpartum weight loss. MCHJ 21(8): 1591-97.

Lebovitz HE (2003). The relationship of obesity to the metabolic syndrome. Int J Clin Prac Supp 134: 18-27.

Lee V, Darney B, Snowden J *et al* (2016). Term elective induction of labour and perinatal outcomes in obese women: retrospective cohort study. BJOG 123(2): 271–78.

Leung T, Stuart O, Suen S *et al* (2011). Comparison of perinatal outcomes of shoulder dystocia alleviated by different type and sequence of manoeuvres: a retrospective review. BJOG 118: 985-90.

Levine EM, Delfinado LN, Locher S *et al* (2021). Reducing the cesarean delivery rate. EJOGRB 262: 155-59.

Lewis P (2013). Room 101 – The only place for fetal monitoring in labour. British Journal of Midwifery 21(6): 386.

Lim S, Harrison C, Callander E *et al* (2022). Addressing obesity in preconception, pregnancy, and postpartum: A review of the literature. Curr Obes Rep 11(4): 405-14.

Lindqvist PG, Bremme K, Hellgren M *et al* (2011). Efficacy of obstetric thromboprophylaxis and long-term risk of recurrence of venous thromboembolism. AOGS 90: 648–53.

Little J, Nugent R & Vangaveti V (2019). Influence of maternal obesity on Bishop Score and failed induction of labour: A retrospective cohort study in a regional tertiary centre. ANZJOG 59: 243-50.

Liu B, Xu G, Sun Y *et al* (2019). Association between maternal pre-pregnancy obesity and preterm birth according to maternal age and race or ethnicity. Lancet Diab Endocrinol 7: 707-14.

Liu J, Wilcox S, Hutto B *et al* (2022). Effects of a lifestyle intervention on postpartum weight retention among women with elevated weight. Obesity (Silver Spring) 30(7): 1370-79.

Logel C, Stinson DA & Brochu PM (2015). Weight loss is not the answer: a well-being solution to the "obesity problem". Social and Personality Psychology Compass 9(12): 678-95.

Lu MY, Blanchard CT, Ausbeck EB *et al* (2021). Evaluation of a risk-stratified, heparin-based, obstetric thromboprophylaxis protocol. O&G 138(4): 530-38.

Lukasse M, Rowe R, Townend J *et al* (2014). Immersion in water for pain relief and the risk of intrapartum transfer among low risk nulliparous women: secondary analysis of the Birthplace national prospective cohort study. BMC P&C 14:60.

Lupton D (2012). Fat (Shortcuts). Hoboken: Taylor and Francis.

Ma'ayeh M & Costantine MM (2020). Prevention of preeclampsia. Seminars Fet Neonat Med 25(5): 101-23.

Mahase E (2021). Stop using body mass index as measure of health, say MPs. BMJ 2021: 373: n941.

Marchi J, Berg M, Dencker A *et al* (2015). Risks associated with obesity in pregnancy, for the mother and baby: a systematic review of reviews. Obes Rev 16(8): 621-38.

Marmot M (2020). Health equity in England: the Marmot review 10 years on. BMJ 368: m693.

Martin KE, Grivell RM, Yelland LN *et al* (2015). The influence of maternal BMI and gestational diabetes on pregnancy outcome. Diabetes Res Clin Pract 108(3): 508-13.

Martis R, Crowther CA, Shepherd E *et al* (2018). Treatments for women with gestational diabetes mellitus: an overview of Cochrane systematic reviews. Cochrane Database Syst Rev 2018(8): CD012327.

Maude RM & Kim M (2020). Getting into the water: a prospective observational study of water immersion for labour and birth at a New Zealand District Health Board. BMC P&C 20: 312.

Mayefske M (2021). Fat Birth. Confident, strong and empowered pregnancy at every size. (n.p.).

McParlin C, Hodson K, Barnes AC *et al* (2019). Views, experience and adherence among pregnant women with gestational diabetes participating in a weight loss study (WELLBABE). Diabet Med 36(2): 195-202.

Middleton P, Shepherd E, Gomersall JC *et al* (2021). Venous thromboembolism prophylaxis for women at risk during pregnancy and the early postnatal period. Cochrane Database Syst Rev 2021(3): CD001689.

Milner J & Arezina J (2018). The accuracy of ultrasound estimation of fetal weight in comparison to birth weight: A systematic review. Ultrasound. 26(1): 32-41.

Minadeo M & Pope L (2022). Weight-normative messaging predominates on TikTok—A qualitative content analysis. PLoS ONE 17(11): e0267997.
Ministry of Health (2021). Annual Data Explorer 2020/21: New Zealand Health Survey. bit.ly/3KVXGI4
Mismetti P, Laporte S, Darmon JY *et al* (2001). Meta-analysis of low molecular weight heparin in the prevention of venous thromboembolism in general surgery. Br J Surg 88: 913–30.
Modder J & Fitzsimons KJ (2010) CMACE/RCOG Joint Guidance. Management of women with obesity in pregnancy. bit.ly/43M20Bg
Mollard E & Cottrell C (2023). Lifestyle and the hypertensive disorders of pregnancy in nulliparous women in the United States: a secondary data analysis of the nuMom2b. BMC P&C 23: 201.
Mone F, Harrity C, Toner B *et al* (2014). Predicting why women have elective repeat cesarean deliveries and predictors of successful vaginal birth after cesarean. IJGO 126(1): 67-69.
Muennig P, Jia H, Lee R *et al* (2008). I think therefore I am: perceived ideal weight as a determinant of health. Am J Pub Hlth 98(3): 501-06.
Muktabhant B, Lawrie TA, Lumbiganon P *et al* (2015). Diet or exercise, or both, for preventing excessive weight gain in pregnancy. Cochrane Database Syst Rev 2015(6): CD007145.
Mulherin K, Miller YD & Barlow FK (2013). Weight stigma in maternity care: women's experiences and care providers' attitudes. BMC P&C 19. doi: 10.1186/1471-2393-13-19.
Nagl M, Linde K, Stepan H *et al* (2015). Obesity and anxiety during pregnancy and postpartum: A systematic review. J Affect Dis 186: 293-305.
Nagpal TS, Salas XR, Vallis M *et al* (2022). Exploring weight bias internalization in pregnancy. BMC P&C 22(605).
Nakimuli A, Chazara O, Byamugisha J *et al* (2014). Pregnancy, parturition and preeclampsia in women of African ancestry. AJOG 210(6): 510-20.e1.
Neel A & Teale G (2019). Considerations for the obese obstetric patient. O&G Magazine 21(3).
Neel A, Cunningham CE & Teale GR (2021). A routine third trimester growth ultrasound in the obese pregnant woman does not reliably identify fetal growth abnormalities: A retrospective cohort study. ANZJOG 61: 116-22.
NHS England (2021). Screening for Down's syndrome, Edwards' syndrome and Patau's syndrome: non-invasive prenatal testing (NIPT). Operational guidance to support the offer of NIPT. London: NHS England.
NICE (2010) Weight management before, during and after pregnancy. Public health guideline PH27. London: NICE.

NICE (2019a). Antenatal care for uncomplicated pregnancies. Clinical guideline CG62. London: NICE.
NICE (2019b). Hypertension in pregnancy. Quality Standard QS35. London: NICE.
NICE (2020). Diabetes in pregnancy: management from preconception to the postnatal period. NICE Guideline NG3. London: NICE.
NICE (2022). Intrapartum care for healthy women and babies. Clinical guideline CG 90. London: NICE.
Nyman VMK, Prebensen ÃK & Flensner GEM (2010). Obese women's experiences of encounters with midwives and physicians during pregnancy and childbirth. Midwifery 26(4): 424-29.
O'Brien TE, Ray JG, Chan WS (2003). Maternal body mass index and the risk of preeclampsia: systematic overview. Epidemiology 14(3): 368-74.
OBS Cymru Quality and Safety Sub Group of Maternity Network Wales & Macgillivray E (2017). All Wales Guideline Prevention and Management of Postpartum Haemorrhage. Cardiff: OBS Cymru.
Ochner CN, Barrios DM, Lee CD *et al* (2013). Biological mechanisms that promote weight regain following weight loss in obese humans. Physiol Behav 15(120): 106-13.
Odent M (1994). Birth reborn: what childbirth should be. 2nd edition. London: Souvenir Press.
O'Dwyer V, Farah N, Hogan J *et al* (2012). Timing of screening for gestational diabetes mellitus in women with moderate and severe obesity. AOGS 91(4): 447-51.
Ogden C, NCHS, and National Health and Nutrition Examination Survey (2015) Prevalence of obesity among adults and youth: United States, 2011-2014. Centers for Disease Control: National Center for Health Statistics.
Ojalehto E, Zhan Y, Jylhävä J *et al* (2023). Genetically and environmentally predicted obesity in relation to cardiovascular disease: a nationwide cohort study. eClinicalMedicine bit.ly/403Hqcu
Olsen O & Clausen JA (2023). Planned hospital birth compared with planned home birth for pregnant women at low risk of complications. Cochrane Database Syst Rev 3(3): CD000352.
Østborg TB, Sande RK, Kessler J (2022), TM. Put your weight behind it—Effect of body mass index on the active second stage of labour: A retrospective cohort study. BJOG 129(13): 2166-74.
Panda S, Begley C & Daly D (2022) Clinicians' views of factors influencing decision-making for CS for first-time mothers—A qualitative descriptive study. PLoS ONE 17(12): e0279403.
Parker L & Bero L (2022). Managing risk from conflicts of interest in guideline development committees. BMJ. 6(379): e072252.
Perry A, Stephanou A & Rayman MP (2022). Dietary factors that affect the risk of pre-eclampsia. BMJ Nutr Prev Health. 5(1): 118-33.

Pettersen-Dahl A, Murzakanova G, Sandvik L *et al* (2018). Maternal body mass index as a predictor for delivery method. AOGS 97: 212- 218.
Pickens C, Gibbs M, Kramer MR *et al* (2018). Term elective induction of labor and pregnancy outcomes among obese women and their offspring. O&G 131(1): 12–22.
Polic A, Curry TL & Louis JM (2022). The impact of obesity on the management and outcomes of postpartum hemorrhage. Am J Perinatol 39(6): 652-57.
Politi S, Mastroroberto L & Ghi P (2023). The time has come for a paradigm shift in obstetrics' medico-legal litigations. EJOGRB 284: 1-4.
Poobalan AS, Aucott LS, Gurung T *et al* (2009). Obesity as an independent risk factor for elective and emergency caesarean delivery in nulliparous women – systematic review and meta-analysis of cohort studies. Obesity Reviews 10: 28-35.
Poorolajal J & Jenabi E (2016). The association between body mass index and preeclampsia: a meta-analysis. J Matern Fetal Neonatal Med 29: 3670–76.
Pressman K & Običan S (2023). Congenital anomalies in women with Obesity. Curr Ob Gyn Rep doi.org/10.1007/s13669-023-00352-z
Preusting I, Brumley J, Odibo L *et al* (2017). Obesity as a predictor of delayed lactogenesis II. J Hum Lact 33(4): 684-91.
Prusova K, Tyler A, Churcher L & Lokugamage AU (2014). Royal College of Obstetricians and Gynaecologists guidelines: How evidence-based are they? 1-6. JOG 34(8): 706–11.
Public Health England (2019). Health of women before and during pregnancy: health behaviours, risk factors and inequalities. bit.ly/3zVm4Dy
Public Health England (2020a). Maternity high impact area: Supporting healthy weight before and between pregnancies. bit.ly/3MG0qL4
Public Health England (2020b). Overweight Adults. bit.ly/3GGJ6lj
Puhl RM & Heuer CA (2010). Obesity stigma: important considerations for public health. AJPH 100(6): 1019-28.
Ramji N, Quinlan J, Murphy P *et al* (2016). The Impact of Maternal Obesity on Breastfeeding. JOGC 38(8): 703-11.
Ramji N, Challa S, Murphy PA *et al* (2018). A comparison of breastfeeding rates by obesity class. JMFNM 31(22): 3021-26.
RANZCOG (2022). Management of Obesity in Pregnancy. Victoria: RANZCOG. bit.ly/42bbR1c
Ravid E, Salzer L, Arnon L *et al* (2018) Is there an association between maternal anxiety propensity and pregnancy outcomes? BMC P&C 18(1): 1-6.
RCOG (2012). Green top Guideline 42: Shoulder Dystocia. London: RCOG.
RCOG (2015). Reducing the risk of venous thromboembolism during

pregnancy and the puerperium. Green-top Guideline 37a. London: RCOG.
RCOG (2018). Care of women with obesity in pregnancy. Green-top Guideline 72. London: RCOG.
RCOG (2021). Gestational diabetes. Patient information leaflet. London: RCOG.
RCOG (2022). Pre-eclampsia. Patient information leaflet. London: RCOG.
Reed R (2022). Gestational Diabetes: beyond the label. bit.ly/3GHoc5A
Relph S, NMPA Project Team (2021). NHS maternity care for women with a body mass index of 30 kg/m^2 or above: Births between 1 April 2015 and 31 March 2017 in England, Wales and Scotland. London: RCOG.
Relph S, Ong M, Vieira MC *et al* (2020). Perceptions of risk and influences of choice in pregnant women with obesity. An evidence synthesis of qualitative research. PLoS ONE 15(1): e0227325.
Research and Markets (2021). Global Weight Loss Products and Services Market 2021-2026. bit.ly/3MFvj2i
Rietveld AL, Teunissen PW, Kazemier BM *et al* (2017). Effect of interpregnancy interval on the success rate of trial of labor after cesarean. J Perinatol 37(11): 1192-96.
Rodrigues PB, Zambaldi CF, Cantilino A et al (2016). Special features of high-risk pregnancies as factors in development of mental distress: a review. Trends Psychiatry Psychother 38(3): 136-140.
Ronnberg A, Hanson U, Ostlund I *et al* (2016). Effects on postpartum weight retention after antenatal lifestyle intervention – a secondary analysis of a randomized controlled trial. AOGS 95: 999–1007.
Rossi AC, Mullin P & Prefumo F (2013). Prevention, management, and outcomes of macrosomia: a systematic review of literature and meta-analysis. Obs Gyn Surv 68(10): 702-09.
Rotchell YE, Cruickshank JK, Gay MP *et al* (1998). Barbados low dose aspirin study in pregnancy: a randomised trial for the prevention of pre-eclampsia and its complications. BJOG 105(3): 286-92.
Rothman KJ (2008). BMI-related errors in the measurement of obesity. Int J Obes 32 Suppl 3: S56-9.
Rottenstreich A, Karlin A, Kalish Y *et al* (2020). Factors associated with women's adherence to postpartum thromboprophylaxis. J Thromb 49(2): 304-11.
Rowe R, Knight M, Kurinczuk JJ *et al* (2018). Outcomes for women with BMI >35kg/m^2 admitted for labour care to alongside midwifery units in the UK: A national prospective cohort study using the UK Midwifery Study System (UKMidSS). PLoS One 4:13(12): e0208041.
Rubino F, Puhl R, Cummings DE *et al* (2020). Joint international consensus statement for ending stigma of obesity. Nat Med 26: 485–97.

Ruhstaller K (2015). Induction of labor in the obese patient. Semin Perinatol 39(6): 437-40.

Ruhstaller KE, Elovitz MA, Stringer M *et al* (2017). Obesity and the association with maternal mental health symptoms. JMFNM 30(16): 1897-1901.

Rydahl E, Eriksen L & Juhl M (2019). Effects of induction of labor prior to post-term in low-risk pregnancies: a systematic review. JBI Database System Rev Implement Rep. 17(2): 170-208.

Saeed KBM, Greene RA, Corcoran P *et al* (2017). Incidence of surgical site infection following caesarean section: a systematic review and meta-analysis protocol BMJ Open 7: e013037.

Sandall J, Soltani H, Gates S *et al* (2016). Midwife-led continuity models versus other models of care for childbearing women. Cochrane Database Syst Rev 2016(4): CD004667.

Sandall J, Tribe RM, Avery L *et al* (2018). Short-term and long-term effects of caesarean section on the health of women and children. Lancet 392(10155): 1349-57.

Sanders J, Hunter B & Warren L (2016). A wall of information? Exploring the public health component of maternity care in England. Midwifery 34: 253-60.

Saqlain M, Khalid M, Fiaz M *et al* (2022). Risk variants of obesity associated genes demonstrate BMI raising effect in a large cohort. PLoS ONE 17(9): e0274904.

Sartwelle TP & Johnston JC (2018). Continuous electronic fetal monitoring during labor: A critique and a reply to contemporary proponents. Surj J (NY) 04(01): e23-e28.

Scarf VL, Rossiter C, Vedam S *et al* (2018). Maternal and perinatal outcomes by planned place of birth among women with low-risk pregnancies in high-income countries: A systematic review and meta-analysis. Midwifery 62: 240-255.

Schieve LA, Cogswell ME, Scanlon KS *et al* (2000). Prepregnancy body mass index and pregnancy weight gain: associations with preterm delivery: the NMIHS Collaborative Study Group. O&G 96(2): 194-200.

Schummers L, Hutcheon JA, Bodnar LM *et al* (2015). Risk of adverse pregnancy outcomes by prepregnancy body mass index: a population-based study to inform prepregnancy weight loss counseling. O&G 125(1): 133-43.

Sebire NJ, Jolly M, Harris JP *et al* (2001). Maternal obesity and pregnancy outcome: a study of 287,213 pregnancies in London. Int J of Obesity 25: 1175-82.

Seimon RV, Natasha N, Schneuer FJ *et al* (2022). Maternal and neonatal outcomes of women with gestational diabetes and without specific medical conditions: an Australian population-based study comparing induction of labor with expectant management. ANZJOG 62(4):525-35.

Shipton E, Meloncelli N, D'Emden M *et al* (2022). Gestational diabetes screening from the perspective of consumers: Insights from early in the COVID-19 pandemic and opportunities to optimise experiences. ANZJOG doi.org/10.1111/ajo.13600

Slack E, Best KE, Rankin J *et al* (2019). Maternal obesity classes, preterm and post-term birth: a retrospective analysis of 479,864 births in England. BMC P&C 19: 434.

Small K (2023) Do bigger women benefit from intrapartum CTG monitoring? bit.ly/3oc8usw

Small KA, Sidebotham M, Fenwick J *et al* (2020). Intrapartum cardiotocograph monitoring and perinatal outcomes for women at risk: Literature review. Women and Birth 33(5): 411-18.

Stalheim AM, Iversen MM, Jenum AK *et al* (2023). Seasonal variation in gestational diabetes mellitus among women in Norway: a national population-based study. BMJ Open 13:e063725.

Stothard KJ, Tennant PW, Bell R *et al* (2009). Maternal overweight and obesity and the risk of congenital anomalies: a systematic review and meta-analysis. JAMA 301(6): 636-50.

Strings S (2015). Obese Black Women as "Social Dead Weight": Reinventing the "Diseased Black Woman." Signs 41(1): 107-30.

Strings S (2019). Fearing the Black Body: The Racial Origins of Fat Phobia. New York University Press.

Stunkard A & Mclaren-Hume (1959). The results of treatment for obesity: a review of the literature and report of a series. AMA Arch Intern Med 103(1): 79-85.

Teale G (2020). Managing pregnancies complicated by obesity. O&G magazine 22(3).

Teufel F, Seiglie JA, Geldsetzer P *et al* (2021) Body-mass index and diabetes risk in 57 low-income and middle-income countries: a cross-sectional study of nationally representative, individual-level data in 685 616 adults. The Lancet 398 (10296): 238-248.

Thorbjörnsdottir KE, Karlsen IE, Dahl B *et al* (2020). "Talk to me, not at me": obese women's experiences of birth and their encounter with birth attendants. Int J Qual Stud Hlth Well-being 15(1): 1845286.

Tieu J, McPhee AJ, Crowther CA *et al* (2017). Screening for gestational diabetes mellitus based on different risk profiles and settings for improving maternal and infant health. Cochrane Database Syst Rev 2017(8): CD007222.

Tomiyama AJ, Carr D, Granberg EM *et al* (2018). How and why weight stigma drives the obesity 'epidemic' and harms health. BMC Med 16(1): 123.

Townsend R, Khalil A, Premakumar Y *et al* (2019). Prediction of pre-eclampsia: review of reviews. Ultrasound Obstet Gynecol 54: 16-27.

Treasure J & Ambwani S (2021). Addressing weight stigma and anti-obesity rhetoric in policy changes to prevent eating disorders. Lancet 398(10294): 7-8.
Tyldesley-Marshall N, Greenfield SM, Parretti HM *et al* (2021). The experiences of postnatal women and healthcare professionals of a brief weight management intervention embedded within the national child immunisation programme. BMC P&C 21(1): 462.
Tyson K, Teale G, Vasilevski V *et al* (2022). A dedicated antenatal clinic for pregnant women with morbid and super-obesity: Patient characteristics, outcomes, perceptions and lessons learnt from establishing the DIAMOND clinic. ANZJOG 62: 635-42.
Tzadikevitch-Geffen K, Melamed N, Aviram A *et al* (2021). Neonatal outcome by planned mode of delivery in women with a body mass index of 35 or more: a retrospective cohort study. BJOG 128(5): 900-06.
UK Parliament (2021). Changing the perfect picture: an inquiry into body image. bit.ly/3ZZTjzT
Ulfsdottir H, Saltvedt S & Georgsson S (2018). Waterbirth in Sweden – a comparative study. AOGS 97: 341– 48.
US Preventive Services Task Force (USPSTF); Davidson KW, Barry MJ *et al* (2021). Screening for Gestational Diabetes: US Preventive Services Task Force Recommendation Statement. JAMA 326(6): 531-38.
Vadiveloo M & Mattei J (2017). Perceived Weight Discrimination and 10-Year Risk of Allostatic Load Among US Adults. Ann Behav Med. 51(1): 94-104. Erratum in: Ann Behav Med 51(1): 105.
Vats H, Saxena R, Sachdeva MP *et al* (2021). Impact of maternal pre-pregnancy body mass index on maternal, fetal and neonatal adverse outcomes in the worldwide populations: A systematic review and meta-analysis. Obes Res Clin Pract 15: 536–45.
Vena F, D'Ambrosio V, Paladini V *et al* (2022). Risk of neural tube defects according to maternal body mass index: a systematic review and meta-analysis. JMFNM 35(25): 7296-7305.
Vestergaard AL, Christensen M, Andreasen MF *et al* (2023). Vitamin D in pregnancy – a randomised controlled trial identifying associations and mechanisms linking maternal Vitamin D deficiency to placental dysfunction and adverse pregnancy outcomes. BMC P&C 23: 177.
Vincent S, Czuzoj-Shulman N, Spence AR *et al* (2018). Effect of pre-pregnancy body mass index on respiratory-related neonatal outcomes in women undergoing elective cesarean prior to 39 weeks. J Perinat Med 46(8): 905-12.
Vinter CA, Jensen DM, Ovesen P *et al* (2014). Postpartum weight retention and breastfeeding among obese women from the randomized controlled Lifestyle in Pregnancy (LiP) trial. AOGS 93(8): 794-801.
Vireday P (2008). The business of scare tactics. bit.ly/3N01kSO

Vireday P (2010). The fat vagina theory: "soft tissue dystocia." bit.ly/3o5YxwS
Vireday P (2017a). Preventing cesarean complications in high BMI women. bit.ly/3KUSmEJ
Vireday P (2017b). Intuitive eating and postpartum weight. bit.ly/3oaZDYl
Walker R, Bennett C, Blumfield M *et al* (2018). Attenuating pregnancy weight gain - what works and why: a systematic review and meta-analysis. Nutrients 10(7): 944.
Wallstrom T, Bjorklund J, Frykman J *et al* (2018). Induction of labor after one previous cesarean section in women with an unfavorable cervix: A retrospective cohort study. PLoS One 13(7): e0200024.
Walsh D (2012). Evidence and skills for normal labour and birth: a guide for midwives. 2nd edition. Abingdon: Routledge.
Wang Z, Wang P, Liu H (2013). Maternal adiposity as an independent risk factor for pre-eclampsia: a meta-analysis of prospective cohort studies. Obes Rev 14: 508–21.
Weiss JL, Malone FD, Emig D *et al* (2004). Obesity, obstetric complications and cesarean delivery rate - a population-based screening study. AJOG 190(4): 1091-97.
WHO (1995). Physical status: the use and interpretation of anthropometry. Report of a WHO Expert Consultation: World Health Organization Technical Report, Series number 854. Geneva: World Health Organization.
WHO (2004). Appropriate body-mass index for Asian populations and implications for policy and intervention strategies. Lancet 363: 157-63.
WHO (2018). WHO recommendations: induction of labour at or beyond term. Geneva: World Health Organization.
Wickham S (2004). Risk: the game of life. TPM 7(6): 41.
Wickham S (2009). Obesity: naming, blaming and shaming. TPM 12(10): 20-21.
Wickham S (2014). Labour progress myths: why size and age may not be the problem. bit.ly/44mAnOG
Wickham S (2017). Birth outcomes in plus size pregnancy. bit.ly/3NwjAl4
Wickham S (2018). Inducing Labour: making informed decisions. Second edition. Avebury: Birthmoon Creations.
Wickham S (2019a) Group B Strep Explained. Second edition. Avebury: Birthmoon Creations.
Wickham S (2019b). Induction of labour and larger women: what are the consequences? bit.ly/3Oe4jGe
Wickham S (2021a). In Your Own Time: how western medicine controls the start of labour and why this needs to stop. Avebury: Birthmoon Creations.

Wickham S (2021b). Anti-D Explained. Avebury: Birthmoon Creations.
Wickham S (2022). What's Right For Me? Making decisions in pregnancy and childbirth. Avebury: Birthmoon Creations.
Wickham S (2023). Gestational Diabetes. bit.ly/3IJnLbL
Wing RR & Jeffrey RW (1979). Outpatient treatment of obesity: a comparison of methodology and clinical results. Int J Obesity 3(3): 261-79.
Wischnik A, Lehmann KJ, Ziegler M *et al* (1992). [Does the "fatty pelvis" exist? Quantitative computer tomography studies]. Z Geburtshilfe Perinatol. 196(6): 247-52.
Wloch C, Wilson J, Lamagni T *et al* (2012). Risk factors for surgical site infection following caesarean section in England: results from a multicentre cohort study. BJOG 119(11): 1324-33.
Wolfe H, Timofeev J, Tefera E *et al* (2014). Risk of cesarean in obese nulliparous women with unfavorable cervix: elective induction vs expectant management at term. AJOG 211(1): 53.e1–5.
Wolrich J (2021). Food isn't medicine. London: Vermilion.
Woolner AMF & Bhattacharya S (2015). Obesity and stillbirth. Best Pract Res Clin Obstet Gynaecol 29(3): 415-26.
Wray S & Deery R (2008). The Medicalization of Body Size and Women's Healthcare. Health Care for Women Int 29(3): 227–43.
Wu YK & Berry DC (2018). Impact of weight stigma on physiological and psychological health outcomes for overweight and obese adults: A systematic review. JAN 74(5): 1030-42.
Xiao J, Mazurak VC, Olobatuyi TA *et al* (2018). Visceral Adiposity and Cancer Survival: A Review of Imaging Studies. E J Cancer Care 27: e12611.
Zareba P, Wu C, Agzarian J *et al* (2014). Meta-analysis of randomised trials comparing combined compression and anticoagulation with either modality alone for prevention of venous thromboembolism after surgery. Br J Surg 101: 1053–62.
Zeng S, Yang Y, Han C *et al* (2023). Burden and trend of macrosomia and large-for-gestational-age neonates attributable to high pre-pregnancy body mass index in China 2013-2017. Healthcare (Basel) 11(3): 331.
Zhang J, Bricker L, Wray S *et al* (2007). Poor uterine contractility in obese women. BJOG 114: 343-48.
Zhang H, Liu H, Luo S *et al* (2021). Oxytocin use in trial of labor after cesarean and its relationship with risk of uterine rupture in women with one previous cesarean section: a meta-analysis of observational studies. BMC P&C 21(1): 11.
Zhao Y, Flatley C, Kumar S (2017). Intrapartum intervention rates and perinatal outcomes following induction of labour compared to expectant management at term from an Australian perinatal centre. ANZJOG 57(1): 40-48.

Also by Sara Wickham

In Your Own Time: how western medicine controls the start of labour and why this needs to stop

Pregnant women and maternity services are facing an induction epidemic. In this timely book, Dr Sara Wickham demystifies the evidence and highlights the significant discrepancies between guidelines and what we really know about the benefits of supporting women to birth spontaneously. In Your Own Time details how we got to this state and looks at the evidence relating to due dates, 'post-term', older and larger women, suspected big babies, maternal race and more.

Anti-D Explained

Anti-D is a medicine made from blood that is offered to rhesus negative women who may have been exposed to rhesus positive blood, for example as their baby is being born. Anti-D Explained helps parents and professionals to understand the science, the issues and the evidence relating to Anti-D.

Inducing Labour: making informed decisions

Sara's bestselling book explains the process of induction of labour and shares information from research studies, debates and women's, midwives' and doctors' experiences to help women and families get informed and decide what is right for them.

Group B Strep Explained

Explains everything that parents and birth workers need to know about Group B Strep; a common and usually harmless bacteria which can occasionally cause problems for babies. Sara discusses screening, preventative measures, alternatives and wider issues.

Also by Sara Wickham

Vitamin K and the Newborn

Find out everything you need to know about vitamin K; why it's offered to newborn babies, why are there different viewpoints on it and what do parents need to know in order to make the decision that is right for them and their baby?

What's Right For Me? Making decisions in pregnancy and childbirth

The decisions that we make about our childbirth journeys can shape our experiences, health and lives, and those of our families. A guide to the different approaches that exist; offering information, tips and tools to help you make the decisions that are right for you.

Birthing Your Placenta (with Nadine Edwards)

A popular book which helps parents, professionals and others to understand the process and the evidence relating to the birth of the placenta. No matter what kind of birth you are hoping for, this book will help you understand the issues and options.

101 tips for planning, writing and surviving your dissertation

These 101 tips are useful for students at any stage of their academic career. Written in an accessible, friendly style and seasoned with first-hand advice, this book combines sound, practical tips from an experienced academic with reminders of the value of creativity, chocolate and naps in your work.

Printed in Great Britain
by Amazon